Ephedra: What You Have NOT Heard

"At the time Mr. Bechler collapsed from heat stroke, much of the ephedrine he had swallowed was still in his stomach and had not yet entered his bloodstream. [The unabsorbed ephedrine] could not have caused or contributed to Mr. Bechler's death."
– *Forensic pathologist Dr. Michael Baden, former New York City chief medical examiner, in a letter to the Subcommittee on Oversight and Investigations Hearing on Issues Relating to Ephedra-Containing Dietary Supplements, July 23, 2003*

"Her blood alcohol limit was .212, more than twice the legally intoxicated limit in most states. Are these two cases really ephedra deaths?"
– *Dan Burton (R-IN), referring to cases included in the FDA's log of adverse reports against ephedra, of which one described a woman who died after colliding with pole at 90 mph going the wrong way on a one-way street*

"There is no scientific data proving that consumption of ephedra/caffeine combinations for weight loss are unsafe, when consumed in accordance with appropriate warning labels."
– *Carol Boozer, M.D., in testimony to Subcommittee on Oversight and Investigations Hearing on Issues Relating to Ephedra-Containing Dietary Supplements, July 2003*

"The FDA has ample authority to act against supplements that do not provide the full amounts of the nutrients they are labeled as providing. Yet the agency has done almost nothing to use this authority. . . . There is no need to amend DSHEA to increase FDA's authority over such products."
– *Stephen N. McNamara and A. Wes Siegner, Jr. (partners at the law firm of Hyman, Phelps & McNamara, P.C., in Washington, D.C.)*

"The NFL basically scapegoated ephedra. . . . It's stupid. I worry a lot more about all the anti-inflammatories NFL teams hand out."
– *Philadelphia Eagles guard John Welbourn, as quoted in* Sports Illustrated

Ephedra: What You Have NOT Heard

"I am concerned about the apparent lack of scientific data behind the FDA's actions. For the FDA—one of the most important regulatory agencies in government—to use such poor science for a dietary supplement raises warning flags for the other products the agency regulates."
– *House Science Committee Chairman F. James Sensenbrenner, Jr. (R-WI)*

"There's almost a witch hunt going on . . . It hasn't been proven that ephedrine caused his [Bechler's] death. There was probably some milk found in his system, too. Did that cause his death?"
– *David Segui, Baltimore Orioles teammate of Steve Bechler*

"Conservative estimates suggest no greater risk for adverse events [from ephedra] than the risk in the general population."
– *Stephen E. Kimmel, M.D., presenting the findings of a panel at hearings at the Office of Women's Health in August 2000*

"Closer examination of contributing factors related to Mr. Bechler's death reveals that even if Mr. Bechler did consume the supplement, it was probably the least of the contributing factors leading to his death—and it may not have been a factor at all."
– *Statement from Baylor University panel of researchers headed by Richard B. Kreider, Ph.D., regarding the case of Baltimore Orioles pitcher Steve Bechler*

"I would have been better off smoking crack. I would have got a slap on the wrist."
– *Denver Broncos player Lee Flowers, responding to his four-game suspension by the NFL after inadvertently taking a supplement that contained ephedra*

"There was no ephedra in there. There was none of the other stuff that they said was in there that contained ephedra."
– *James Montgomery, attorney for the mother of Northwestern University football player Rashidi Wheeler, referring to the list of items present in Wheeler's locker. Refuting the medical examiner's report that Wheeler died on the practice field of an asthma attack, school officials alleged that Wheeler's death was due to his using some sort of ephedra product.*

Ephedra
Fact & Fiction

How Politics, the Press and
Special Interests Are Targeting
Your Rights to Vitamins,
Minerals and Herbs

Mike Fillon

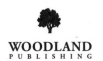

WOODLAND
PUBLISHING

The CIP record for this book is available from the Library of Congress.

For ordering information, contact:
Woodland Publishing, 448 East 800 North, Orem, Utah 84097
(800) 777-2665

The information in this book is for educational purposes only and is not
recommended as a means of diagnosing or treating an illness. All mat-
ters concerning physical and mental health should be supervised by a
health practitioner knowledgeable in treating that particular condition.
Neither the publisher nor author directly or indirectly dispenses medical
advice, nor do they prescribe any remedies or assume any responsibility
for those who choose to treat themselves.

ISBN 1-58054-370-7

Printed in the United States of America
Please visit our website:
www.woodlandpublishing.com

For Emilie

Contents

Foreword

Richard B. Kreider, Ph.D., FACSM, FASEP
Professor & Chair, Exercise & Sport Nutrition Lab
Center for Exercise, Nutrition & Preventive Health
Department of Health, Human Performance & Recreation
Baylor University

ACCORDING TO THE *Nutrition Business Journal,* Americans spent $17.7 billion dollars in 2002 on vitamins, minerals, herbs, specialty supplements, meal replacement, and sports nutrition and weight-loss supplements. Survey research has consistently reported that the majority of respondents (typically 50–80 percent) regularly use some type of dietary supplement such as vitamins, minerals, and herbal products to improve the quality of their diets, enhance general health and well-being, improve performance, and help manage body weight.

Despite the widespread use of dietary supplements among Americans, there currently rages a battle among proponents and opponents of dietary supplements over the safety and efficacy of supplements and the manner in which they are regulated. Although many individuals have a balanced view regarding the controversy, there seem to be two extreme camps. On one hand, there are those who believe that they have a constitutional right to sell or use nutritional supplements they deem beneficial and safe. They don't want the federal government to place undue regulations or restrictions on the development or sale of dietary supplements. Furthermore, they see any attempt to ban or limit the sale of dietary supplements as an infringement on their right to make self-determined health decisions; they also feel that these efforts are usually financially or politically motivated.

On the other hand, there are those who feel that supplements are ineffective, dangerous, and therefore should be heavily restricted or made illegal. They do not feel that current law provides necessary safeguards to ensure the quality or safety of dietary supplements. They see companies who develop and sell dietary supplements as financially motivated charlatans preying on gullible and susceptible consumers. Consequently, they have called on state and federal representatives to place additional regulations and restrictions on the sale of dietary supplements in order to protect the consumer from what they believe are unsafe products. In a number of instances, they have lobbied for an outright ban on the sale of certain dietary supplements and/or a massive overhaul of federal laws governing the dietary supplement industry.

As a scientist who has sought to determine the impact of various nutritional and exercise therapies on health and performance, I have found myself attempting to bridge the gap between credible and incredible claims on both sides of this debate. In this regard, I have challenged companies who develop and sell dietary supplements to conduct research on the safety and efficacy of their products, to fully report results observed to the scientific and medical communities, and to accurately portray results in marketing materials so that consumers can make an informed decision about whether or not to try a particular supplement.

I have also challenged the media, special interest groups, lawyers, and politicians to honestly and accurately reflect the safety and efficacy of dietary supplements to the public. It is my view that comments, policy, and federal regulations regarding dietary supplements should be based on a thorough and honest analysis of the available scientific evidence—not speculation, emotion, unproven hypotheses, or hidden financial or political agendas. Unfortunately, claims about the potential benefits of supplements as well as fears about possible side effects are often overblown by individuals on both sides of this debate. The result is that consumers, sports and health organizations, special interest groups, and politicians are often misinformed about the known safety and efficacy of dietary supplements.

The debate over the safety and efficacy of ephedra is a classic example of how misinformation portrayed in the media and from various special interest groups can cause a political and legal firestorm about a dietary supplement. Although a significant body of scientific evidence indicates that use of synthetic ephedrine or herbal ephedra can safely promote weight loss when used as directed in overweight but otherwise healthy individuals, there have been unprecedented efforts made to see that ephedra is banned for sale in the U.S.

Those in favor of a ban on ephedra point to adverse events voluntarily reported to several poison control centers and adverse event monitoring systems suggesting that some people who took ephedra-containing supplements experienced mild to severe side effects. They also point to several recent deaths among high school, college, and professional athletes who were believed to have taken ephedra-containing supplements as evidence that ephedra is dangerous. This is despite the fact that 1) ephedra has been used as an herbal supplement for thousands of years; 2) an estimated twelve to seventeen million people consume approximately three billion doses of ephedra containing dietary supplements annually; 3) available clinical trials show that ephedrine or ephedra supplementation can be safely used to promote weight loss and/or improve performance in healthy populations; 4) definitive conclusions about the safety of ephedra cannot be made based on available adverse events reported because many are incomplete and reveal a number of additional contributing factors; 5) millions of people in the United States consume over-the-counter cold medications containing pseudoephedrine at equivalent or higher doses than found in dietary supplements; and, 6) the safety profile of ephedra is much better than many over-the-counter and prescription medications.

Those observing this debate have to wonder what commercial, political, or legal interests are behind attempts to ban ephedra, as well as its highly negative portrayals in the media. Further, one has to wonder why such media and political attention has been paid to ephedra when hundreds of thousands of people die each year from using prescription medications, over-the-counter medications, alcohol, and tobacco products.

Ephedra Fact & Fiction is a comprehensive and enlightening overview of the commercial, political, and other dynamics fueling the debate surrounding ephedra and dietary supplement legislation. It provides a fascinating analysis of how the known scientific and medical data has been misrepresented in the media and by special interest groups and politicians, among others. It also exposes apparent conflicts of interest that the pharmaceutical industry, medical community, and politicians involved in the ephedra debate may have and how these conflicts of interest affect the distribution and advertisement of dietary supplements.

The book also provides a concise overview of how the FDA and FTC currently have legal power to remove dangerous products from the market if sufficient scientific evidence shows the product is dangerous and to act against companies who make false advertisements about their products.

It is my hope that this book will enlighten consumers about the commercial and political interests influencing efforts to ban ephedra and change current law regarding the sale and advertisement of dietary supplements. Additionally, I hope that lawmakers will realize that the best way to determine the safety and efficacy of dietary supplements is to conduct research, and therefore increase funding to support this work. This means that that they must realize that additional funding is necessary to help the FDA and FTC enforce existing law on behalf of the American public.

Introduction

In February 2003, Baltimore Orioles pitcher Steve Bechler collapsed and died while at a spring training workout session. Soon enough, it became known that Bechler may have been using an ephedra-based supplement. Almost immediately, newspaper headlines across the country blared: *"Ephedra Kills Baseball Player!"* or similar incendiary words, and pundits, critics and regulators worked themselves into a collective frenzy, many of them calling for tighter regulations and others for an outright ban of the controversial herb.

Did ephedra really kill Steve Bechler? By picking up this book I'm guessing you're not so sure. Well, you're not alone. Over the last several years, ephedra has been both widely hailed for its supposed benefits and roundly criticized for its alleged dangers. Depending on who you talk to, ephedra could be a fantastic weight-loss tool or an evil poison waiting to kill you, just like it did Steve Bechler. No wonder you, like so many, are confused about ephedra.

Before we move on, let's test your knowledge—or confusion—relating to ephedra with this quick quiz:

Question #1: Based on television, newspaper and other media accounts, I believe ephedra is:
  A. Dangerous
  B. Not dangerous
  C. I don't know—I'm befuddled
  D. I find it impossible to form an objective opinion
  E. All of the above

(According to my grading sheet, the correct answer is E.)

Question #2: How many deaths has ephedra caused?
  A. 2
  B. 10
  C. 100
  D. 1,000
  E. Who knows?
  F. Depends on what you read

(Either E or F is the correct answer, although A, B or C could also be right. The sad truth is that no one—not even ephedra's harshest critics—know the answer.)

Question #3: Which has caused the most deaths?
  A. Over-the-counter (OTC) painkillers
  B. Prescription drugs
  C. Ephedra
  D. Aspirin

(The correct answer is B. More than 10,000 Americans are inadvertently killed each year by prescription drugs, and according to the World Health Organization [WHO], prescription medications are the fourth leading cause of death in this country!)

Just What Is Going On Here?

Most everyone is aware that nothing sells newspapers or attracts TV viewers better than a good old-fashioned health scare. When Steve Bechler died, many were quick to blame as the main culprit the ephedra-based fat burning supplement he was taking. Since ephedra was already under fire, it was easy for irresponsible (or lazy, or naïve—take your pick) headline writers to push the ephedra connection, probably causing many folks to rummage through their son's gym bag and their own medicine cabinet searching for the substance.

While there's reason to believe that the ephedra product Bechler was taking, Cytodyne's Xenadrine RFA-1, might have contributed to his death, there were certainly other contributing factors. Because he was some ten to fifteen pounds overweight, and due to pressure from the team to lose this weight and get in shape quickly, Bechler embarked on a low-cal liquid diet. Reports indicate he hadn't eaten any solid foods in two days. He also had a history of borderline high blood pressure and undiagnosed liver abnormalities, and he had experienced episodes of heatstroke earlier in his life. Bechler was also wearing multiple layers of clothing as part of his efforts to sweat off the extra pounds, despite it being quite hot and humid. (We'll discuss Bechler's case at length in Chapter 2.) And needless to say, almost no one is questioning the guidelines of teams and organizations that oversee workout conditions and procedures. Neither is anyone asking if his existing liver condition or history of heatstroke had anything to do with his death.

It's obvious that these and other red flags haven't received the level of publicity the ephedra connection received—not by a long shot. So why has all the heat focused on the ephedra-connection? That is what this book is about.

It's important for us to get something straight. I did not set out to write a book defending ephedra use, nor did I approach the topic ready to denounce it. I did not have—and still do not have—a hidden agenda. When I began the book, I was fully prepared to condemn ephedra if that's what the reams of evidence on my desk showed. Likewise, if I found ephedra to be safe I would trumpet that position.

Everything I read about ephedra, including scores of medical studies, came down on either one side or the other. It seemed to me that everyone had an ax to grind. So where did the truth lie? I suspected that it was somewhere in between, yet no one had staked out that territory. I wanted to know why.

As you'll see, there's more going on here than just hand-wringing over a controversial herb. When you learn about ephedra and the uproar surrounding it, you stumble upon hypocrisy and inconsistency. After all, in a country focusing on the alleged dangers of ephedra, little is said about the painkiller acetaminophen, which has claimed many more lives, or aspartame, which comprises the majority of all the complaints directed to the FDA regarding side effects from drugs, supplements and food additives (some reports put this number as high as 75 percent). Even that relatively benign little staple in everyone's medicine cabinet, aspirin, claims five hundred lives per year. (Before you panic, I'll explain more about that later.) Compare that to the deaths that some say were caused by ephedra (and which occurred over several years, for that matter), and you have to ask yourself why so much fuss is made about ephedra and not things like aspirin or acetaminophen.

We should realize that no matter what we take, whether it be an over-the-counter medication, a prescribed drug or a dietary supplement, there will probably be risks. And yet, we hear the loudest condemnation of and demand for restrictions on a variety of herbs, while we seem to think it's just dandy there's only token regulation for tobacco and alcohol. (And then there's the lovely issue of medicinal marijuana, which reportedly has never killed anyone.) Where is the consistency?

I believe Richard B. Kreider, Ph.D., Professor & Chair, Exercise & Sport Nutrition Laboratory at Baylor University, has it just about right: "Sometimes, we focus on obscure problems—particularly in the media—that in reality have little risk compared to many common activities. The pharmaceutical, alcohol, and tobacco industries have huge political lobbies. The pharmaceutical lobby also has an interest to see supplements that may work as well as some drugs be regulated."

Dr. Kreider points out that even though according to the RAND report—which I cover at length in the book—there may have only been five "sentinel" cases of death related to ephedra use over an approximate ten-year period, we clamor for action against ephedra yet ignore the risks of severe side effects and even death from much more common products—such things as aspirin, acetaminophen, alcohol, tobacco, and others. "It is my view that policy should be based on science not speculation. Unfortunately, in politics the latter often dictates action," says Dr. Kreider, who is also president of the American Society of Exercise Physiologists.

There's no question that at its peak, ephedra was very popular. Although there is no complete tally on how many people have used ephedra, a study of fourteen companies manufacturing and marketing ephedra-containing supplements by the American Herbal Products Association (AHPA) between 1995 and 1999 shows that sales increased 700 percent during that five-year period. In 1995, the reported 425 million servings sold rose to three billion in 1999. According to M. McGuffen of the Department of Health and Human Services at a hearing on safety of ephedra products on August 8, 2000, there were a total of only sixty-six serious adverse events during that period reported by these same companies; or less than ten reports per billion servings sold.

As you'll discover, the issues surrounding ephedra use are quite complex, and they certainly involve money, politics and a lack of common sense. Part of the problem is that ephedra products make fantastic profits for manufacturers promising quick energy and slimmer torsos. These folks will do whatever it takes to defend their markets—just as major pharmaceutical, cigarette and alcohol companies do. In this case, several pharmaceutical companies may be losing consumer dollars to the ephedra manufacturers. Add to that prescription-writing doctors, prescription-filling pharmacists, politicians (a few grandstanding, some dependent on political contributions from lobby groups opposing ephedra), overreacting consumer groups, the media—which vacillates between unquestioned stenography to sensationalism—and you have a chorus of condemnation drowning out reason. Who suffers? You and I, of course, who depend on *all* these groups for honest and accurate information. There's no question outside help is needed. Ideally, this would be provided by the U.S. Food and Drug Administration; that is, if they're up to the task. Not everyone is sure they are.

During my more than fifteen years of science, health and medical writing, I have witnessed all sorts of shenanigans, shoddy interpretation and manipulation when it comes to research. I've seen sound science shouted down by organizations with deep pockets, and sketchy findings overly publicized and underwritten by special interests. Often questionable results are hard to spot, open to interpretation and require some down and dirty "digging." Take the five hundred aspirin deaths I mentioned previously, for example. Many are due to accidental overdose by children and suicidal overdose by adults, and a few are the result of allergic reactions. (*Note:* In 1989, there were 1.28 million ingestion poisonings, of which 5,889 were of aspirin, and ten times more of acetaminophen.) Plus, there's evidence that aspirin actually helps save lives, especially when taken by those with high risk of cardiovascular disease. But if you look at the raw numbers, it looks as if people taking aspirin are keeling over all the time.

It should be obvious that it's very easy to manipulate numbers—to get them to say what you want. Is this what's happening with ephedra? Are opponents putting great weight on the numbers of adverse reactions, while the herb's defenders pooh-pooh them? Possibly. (Believe me, we'll discuss this idea further in later chapters.)

And here's another point. Just as with anything we put in our bodies there are potential risks to using ephedra products, and self-prescribing is never a good idea. Each person's condition is unique and the guidance of an appropriately trained health practitioner should be sought. For example, ephedrine stimulates the central nervous system and increases heart rate. If you already have high blood pressure ephedra could raise it even more.

As I alluded to earlier, it seems that the controversy surrounding ephedra isn't just about the herb. Could it be that ephedra is only the outer ring of this high-stakes archery match? Could it be that the real bullseye—the one politicians, special interests and their allies in the media are aiming for—is DSHEA, the current legislation governing dietary supplements?

While I'm not shy about giving my opinions, in reality, you, the reader and consumer, are judge and jury. I am only the messenger. With that in mind, it's important for you to make a few mental notes as you read:

- Did ephedra's opponents make their case?
- Did ephedra's defenders make their case?
- Is the FDA vigilant enough in their duties not just towards ephedra and dietary supplements—seemingly their favorite targets—but also food and drugs?
- And most importantly, do ephedra's benefits outweigh its risks, or do we still need more studies to determine that?

In the end, if you want the unvarnished facts about ephedra, its safety and effectiveness as a health supplement, you've come to the right place. This book will cut through all the misinformation, confusion and contradiction, and is intended to provide all the correct information you need if you are considering using an ephedra-based product. In other words, this book can help determine if ephedra is right for you.

CHAPTER 1

What Is Ephedra?

EPHEDRA, ALSO KNOWN by the Chinese name *ma huang*, is an adrenaline-like stimulant that affects the heart, nasal passages, lungs and nervous system. Though its use in the U.S. and elsewhere has exploded over the last several years, ephedra has been used for medicinal purposes for over three thousand years, originating in Mongolia and the bordering regions of China. (However, there's no evidence Genghis Khan took it for a boost in energy for an upcoming battle, or members of the Ming Dynasty used it to shed excess weight!)

Ephedra Facts

There are several varieties of ephedra, with *Ephedra sinica* or *Ephedra sinensis* being the most commonly used in nutritional supplement products. In the United States, it's generally just called *ephedra* or by its Chinese name *ma huang* (which means "hemp yellow" because of its color). Botanically, ephedra is more closely related to conifer trees like pine and fir than to familiar flowering plants such as the mints or dandelions.

Harvested in the fall, the broom-like stems from the ephedra shrub are dried, powdered and processed into teas or extracts and shipped all over the world. Although there are several American species, such as *Ephedra nevadensis*—otherwise known as "Mormon tea" or "squaw tea" and used traditionally as a blood purifier—they contain little or no ephedrine, the main active ingredient in the Asian varieties.

The most common historical medicinal use of ephedra was to relieve symptoms of the common cold, asthma and related conditions. In more recent times, synthetic versions of its active ingredients—namely ephedrine and pseudoephedrine—have found world-wide use as ingredients in over-the-counter (OTC) cold and allergy medications. And as you're probably aware, supplement products containing ephedra, ephedrine, and/or pseudoephedrine are now widely used as an aid in losing weight and improving sports performance.

Sounds Good—Then What's the Problem?

The controversy brewing over ephedra has little to do with its traditional use in the treatment of asthma and upper respiratory ailments. Rather it is from the very modern notion that ephedra helps promote weight loss and improvement in athletic performance that this big hubbub has developed. A number of popular weight-loss and energy products include either the whole herb, extracts of the herb, or pure concentrates of its alkaloids, ephedrine and pseudoephedrine. To varying degrees, these products can stimulate the nervous system and increase metabolism by stimulating the thyroid gland, all of which theoretically results in more burned fat. In addition, the ephedra alkaloids also stimulate the heart, cause blood vessels to constrict, and dilate the airways. Manufacturers of diet and energy products claim when blended with "tonic" herbs that help to counteract its side-effects, ephedra is safer to use than other popular stimulants such as coffee, kola nut or guarana, all of which contain caffeine.

While there is evidence ephedra-containing products can help people lose weight and provide energy, there are possible dangerous side effects. Some people using ephedra have reported the following:

- poor digestion
- increased blood pressure
- sleeping difficulties
- nervousness
- anxiety attacks
- general weakness and lethargy
- muscular tremors
- urinary retention (in men with prostatic enlargement)

There are some other problems with ephedra supplements. First, as we just mentioned, some manufacturers add other "tonic" herbs to help counteract some of these negative reactions. We don't know how or if these herbs truly interact, and how they influence the effect of ephedra or its alkaloids. More importantly, many ephedra products also contain caffeine, itself a stimulant which seems to amplify some of ephedra's effects. Finally, as with any medication or supplement, everyone has a different tolerance to ephedra and its main constituents. It is difficult to predict how each individual will respond.

Not only should people with heart disease and hypertension avoid taking ephedrine-containing products, but those with diabetes or hyperthyroidism should use it cautiously as well. Ephedrine can also contract the uterus, meaning it should not be used during pregnancy. (By the way, there are no studies regarding adverse effects on a developing fetus.) And since it passes through the mother's milk to the infant it should not be

What's in a Name?

The term "ephedra" can be confusing. Supplements used for weight loss and sports performance contain "ephedrine alkaloids," naturally occurring compounds found in a variety of plants, with ma huang (*Ephedra sinica* or *E. sinensis*) by far the most common. Ephedra dietary supplements generally contain standardized extracts that have 6-8 percent ephedrine alkaloids and a number of other components which have little influence on the action of the herb.

The most predominant alkoloid in these products is ephedrine (which comprises about 90 percent of the herb's alkaloid content). The rest is made up of pseudoephedrine, and to a much lesser degree, norpseudoephedrine, norephedrine, methylephedrine, and methyl-pseudoephedrine. These slow the absorption of ephedrine from the digestive tract and/or counteract the stimulant effects of the ephedrine in the extracts. Manufacturers are required by law to declare the amount of ephedrine in each serving.

The FDA issued a warning against norephedrine—often called phenylpropanolamine—as a stand-alone extract in November of 2001, stating that it can cause liver damage, bleeding and stroke. In addition, the agency requested that drug companies remove this product from the market.

There is a difference between ephedrine alkaloids and synthetic ephedrine. Synthetic ephedrine and pseudoephedrine, which are used in a number of common cold remedies, are not naturally occurring substances and can be identified on the cold products' label usually with "hydrochloride" attached. Industry standards and some state laws prohibit the use of synthetic ephedrine in ephedra dietary supplement products.

Is there a difference between using products made up of the puri-fied extracts and those using the entire herb? Most likely so. Many scientists and herbalists say using the herb in whole plant form is safer than the alkoloid derivative form. British herbalist Michael McIntyre writes that while pure ephedrine may raise blood pressure, the "whole plant actually reduces blood pressure."

And just a sidenote—unless indicated otherwise, when I use the term "ephedra," I'm usually referring to ephedrine alkaloid formulations made up primarily of ephedrine and pseudoephedrine.

taken when breast-feeding. In addition, ephedra should not be taken with monoamine oxidase (MAO) inhibitors (such as isocarboxazid, phenelzine or tranylcypromine), which limited research shows may heighten the stimulating effects of ephedra.

Animal studies have not demonstrated carcinogenic or mutagenic potential for ephedrine. In addition, the alkaloid is rapidly eliminated from the human body. It has been shown that 88 percent of an oral dose is excreted in the urine within twenty-four hours; 97 percent after forty-eight hours.

Despite the number of side effects listed for purified ephedrine in therapeutic doses, studies show that the whole herb ephedra has a very low toxicity and potential for side effects, especially when used in recommended amounts.

Others Are Concerned

It's not just the government, pharmaceutical companies or lawmakers that are concerned about ephedra. Licensed traditional Chinese medicine (TCM) practitioners worry that the uncontrolled sale of ephedra as a weight-loss/sports supplement to an ill-informed public will cause the herb to be banned or heavily restricted by the FDA, thereby making it unavailable to them for use in their clinics.

Likewise, many herbalists have long argued that ephedra should not be sold for other uses without considering the possible side-effects, as well as clearly defining what kind of person can safely take the herb—and for what ailments or conditions. Other natural practitioners believe manufacturing and advertising products containing ephedra for energy or weight loss is largely irresponsible, and can do nothing but hurt the industry in the long run.

Apparently millions of consumers have been willing to take that risk. Common ephedra-containing products, including Ripped Fuel, Diet Fuel, Metabolife and Thermo Speed continue to fly off the shelves (at least where they're still available). The first question we need to ask is why?

Note: The U.S. Food and Drug Administration (FDA) has an import alert on ephedra extracts, and the herb has been mentioned in Congressional and FDA hearings as a substance about which unsubstantiated claims and documented hazards had occurred in the marketplace. Some manufacturers have been issued warnings by the government. (See Exhibits 1 and 2.) By the way, when I first read these letters, I thought I understood why the government was alarmed over public safety and ephedra. But as I found out—and you will too in a later chapter—HHS took some liberties with the facts regarding safety in general and the RAND report in particular.

Exhibit 1

HHS Acts to Reduce Safety Concerns Associated with Dietary Supplements Containing Ephedra
Fact Sheet
February 28, 2003

TODAY'S ACTION

The Department of Health and Human Services (HHS) today reported on new evidence, including a study by the RAND Corporation, suggesting that dietary supplements containing ephedra may present significant or unreasonable risks as currently marketed, and announced a series of actions designed to protect Americans from these risks. Announced actions by the Food and Drug Administration (FDA) included:

• Seeking rapid public comment on the new evidence on health risks associated with ephedra, to establish an up-to-date public record as quickly as possible to support any appropriate new restrictions on ephedra-containing products.
• Seeking rapid public comment on whether the currently available evidence and medical literature present a "significant or unreasonable risk of illness or injury" from dietary supplements containing ephedra. This is the standard that must be met under the Dietary Supplement Health and Education Act for the government to take regulatory action on ephedra.
• Seeking rapid comment on a strong new warning label on any ephedra products that continue to be marketed. The proposed label warns about reports of serious adverse events after use of ephedra, including heart attack, seizure, stroke, and death; cautions that the risk can increase with the dose, with strenuous exercise, and with other stimulants such as caffeine; specifies certain groups (such as women who are pregnant or breast feeding and persons under 18) who should not use these products; and lists other diseases, such as heart disease and high blood pressure, that should rule out the use of ephedrine alkaloids.
• Issuing a set of warning letters against ephedra products making

unsubstantiated claims about sports performance enhancement. The RAND study found only minimal scientific evidence in support of such health claims.

NEW RAND CORPORATION STUDY

The RAND study, commissioned by the National Institutes of Health and released today, reviewed recent evidence on the risks and benefits of ephedra and ephedrine. The study found limited evidence of an effect of ephedra on short-term weight loss, and minimal evidence of an effect on performance enhancement in certain physical activities. It also concluded that ephedra is associated with higher risks of mild to moderate side effects such as heart palpitations, psychiatric and upper gastrointestinal effects, and symptoms of autonomic hyperactivity such as tremor and insomnia, especially when it is taken with other stimulants. The study reviewed over 16,000 adverse events reported after ephedra use and found about 20 "sentinel events" including heart attack, stroke, and death that occurred in the absence of other contributing factors. In conjunction with other recent studies of serious adverse events involving persons taking ephedra, the RAND study adds significantly to the evidence suggesting that ephedra as currently marketed may be associated with unreasonable safety risks.

Food and Drug Administration
Rockville, MD 20857
5100 Paint Branch Parkway
College Park, Maryland 20740

Exhibit 2

This letter is representative of the letters that will be issued by the agency today, February 28, 2003.

WARNING LETTER

VIA OVERNIGHT DELIVERY
Bryan Green
1-supplements.net
c/o Powerhouse Supplements
576 Glenrose Lane
Cincinnati, OH 45244

Dear Mr. Green:

The Food and Drug Administration (FDA) has reviewed your web site at the address: http://www.1-supplements.net. This review shows what we believe to be violations of the Federal Food, Drug, and Cosmetic Act (the Act) in the labeling of your products Thermbuterol, Gut Cutter, Dymetadrine Xtreme, and 3-Andro Xtreme. You can find the Act and the dietary supplement labeling regulations through links on FDA's Internet home page at: http://www.fda.gov.

Under the Act, dietary supplement labeling may include claims about the supplement's effect on the structure or a function of the human body. To be permissible under the Act, these "structure/function" claims must be truthful and may not be misleading.

The labeling of Thermbuterol, Gut Cutter, Dymetadrine Xtreme, and 3-Andro Xtreme bears structure/function claims that include the following:

- Thermbuterol: "build muscle fast," "enhancing your body's own muscle-building," and "increasing your lean muscle mass by enhancing your body's own muscle-building..."
- Gut Cutter: "feel totally powerful," and "...bodybuilding compound."
- Dymetadrine Xtreme: "strength supplementation," "not only are

you stronger and can train with ultra high intensity," "preserves lean muscle mass," and "supporting lean muscle mass growth."
• 3-Andro Xtreme: "will also help increase strength instantly."

Based on the scientific data available to us, we do not believe that these claims are substantiated. If these claims do not have an adequate scientific basis, they are false or misleading and cause your products to be misbranded within the meaning of Sections 403(a)(1) and 403(r)(6)(B) of the Act. Section 301(a) of the Act prohibits the introduction or delivery for introduction into interstate commerce of any food, including a dietary supplement, that is misbranded. Section 301(k) of the Act prohibits the doing of any act with respect to a food, including a dietary supplement, if such act is done while such article is held for sale (whether or not the first sale) after shipment in interstate commerce and results in such article being misbranded. If you have data which you believe substantiates your claims, please share it with us within fifteen (15) working days of your receipt of this letter.

In addition, except for health claims authorized by FDA, claims that a dietary supplement is intended to prevent, diagnose, mitigate, treat, or cure a disease (disease claims), may cause the supplement to be an unapproved new drug. The Act prohibits the introduction of unapproved new drugs into interstate commerce. If you are making disease claims for Thermbuterol, Gut Cutter, Dymetadrine Xtreme, or 3-Andro Xtreme, please be aware that these claims may violate the Act and subject you or the products to regulatory action without further notice.

This letter is not an all-inclusive review of your web site and the products that your firm markets. It is your responsibility to ensure that all products marketed by your firm comply with the Act and its implementing regulations.

The Act authorizes the seizure of illegal products and injunctions against the manufacturers and distributors of those products. You should take prompt action to correct any violations identified in this letter. Failure to do so may result in enforcement action without further notice.

Please advise this office, in writing and within fifteen working days of receipt of this letter, as to the specific steps that you have taken to correct any violations and to assure that similar violations do not occur. If corrective action cannot be completed with fifteen working days, state the reason for the delay and the time within which the corrections will be made.

Any reply should be sent to the attention of Compliance Officer Quyen Tien at the above address.

Sincerely yours,

Joseph R. Baca
Director
Office of Compliance
Center for Food Safety and Applied Nutrition

CHAPTER 2

The Quest for the Quick Fix and an Added Edge

STEVE BECHLER had high hopes of making the Baltimore Orioles opening day roster. Problem was, the twenty-three-year-old needed to shed between ten and fifteen pounds quickly to improve his chances of making the squad. Instead of making the team, he ended up in the morgue.

Toxicology reports released soon after he died showed that the diet supplement Cytodyne's Xenadrine RFA-1, which contains ephedrine, was present in his system. While the official cause of his death was heatstroke, there is still considerable speculation about the role ephedra played in his death.

Here's why. Shortly after he performed the autopsy, Broward County, Florida medical examiner Dr. Joshua Perper said in his official report that the toxicology analysis "revealed significant amounts of ephedrine" in Bechler's blood, along with smaller amounts of two other stimulants, pseudoephedrine and caffeine. The amount he found is consistent with taking three tablets of the weight-loss supplement Xenadrine.

However, the autopsy—and the investigation into his

death—showed other very pertinent and revealing facts. First, Bechler had virtually no food or liquid in his gastrointestinal tract. He also wore extra layers of clothing to induce extra sweating, which in the Florida heat actually impedes sweat evaporation and reduces cooling. As a result, his self-imposed hypohydration (less than normal total body water) negatively affected his thermoregulatory responses, resulting in sweating, shivering, a rise in heart rate, an extremely high core temperature (reports say he collapsed with a core temperature reportedly of 106°F before being removed from the field) and a decrease in overall performance. Plus, some teammates said he took much more of the Xenadrine product than is recommended—which also elevates heart rate—and probably degraded his condition.

During the investigation of his death, Bechler's teammates reported that he was listless during practice—typical telltale signs of dehydration and heat exhaustion. One report stated he was able to complete only 60 percent of the team workout two days before he died.

To top it off, Bechler suffered from hypertension and liver problems, and had a prior history of heat illness episodes while in high school, all of which only increased the possibility for tragedy.

In response to the public uproar surrounding Bechler's death and the alleged link to ephedra, researchers from Baylor University, led by Richard B. Kreider, Ph.D., Professor & Chair, Exercise & Sport Nutrition Laboratory, released a statement that included their observations and interpretation of what happened to Mr. Bechler.

In addition to the points I've already raised, the Baylor researchers also said the media was guilty of over-sensationalizing the dangers of ephedra use:

"Unfortunately, these media reports may mislead some to conclude that simply prohibiting athletes from taking ephedra supplements will eliminate the risk of heat fatalities," wrote the Baylor University team. Instead, they say, those in charge should be stressing the importance of properly educating athletes, coaches and athletic trainers about the risks of training in hot and humid environments when participants are poorly conditioned, have not acclimatized to the heat and humidity, have engaged in dehydration practices, and/or have questionable medical histories.

"It seems that Major League Baseball and others want to blame ephedra for the death of Mr. Bechler, rather than admit that they may have been negligent in screening, conditioning, and supervising their athletes," wrote the Baylor researchers. "Closer examination of contributing factors related to Mr. Bechler's death reveals that even if Mr. Bechler did consume the supplement, it was probably the least of the contributing factors leading to his death—*and it may not have been a factor at all*" (emphasis is mine).

Is Ephedra Safe?

Since this is the main thrust of the book, we'll be examining this critical issue from various angles and viewpoints throughout. For now, let's just say that suppliers of ephedra products, most experts in alternative medicine and herbalism, and even some "conventional" health experts, believe that when used as directed, ephedra is safe. On the opposing side, the Food and Drug Administration (FDA) says it has compiled a list of over 800 adverse events for ephedra, including heart attack, stroke, tremors, insomnia, and death. One report lists at least seventeen deaths due to supplements containing ephedra.

Here's a list of some of the statements made and actions taken by organizations and entities in response to the ephedra "scare":

• The American Heart Association says the supplement should be banned, saying it does more harm than good.

- In April 2003, The American Society of Health-System Pharmacists (ASHP) urged the FDA to ban the sale of dietary supplements containing ephedra because of significant risks to public health. ASHP warned the labeling changes proposed by the FDA will not protect the public from the dangers of these products.
- A study by the RAND Corporation reports two deaths, four heart attacks, and nine strokes among 16,000 adverse event reports.
- Other research, appearing in the journal *Annals of Internal Medicine* in 2003, shows ephedra is responsible for 64 percent of all adverse reactions reported to Poison Centers from herb use, although it accounts for less than 1 percent of such supplements sold.
- In March 2003, Senator Jackie Speier introduced a law to ban diet supplements containing ephedra in California.
- In March 2003, the editors of the *Journal of the American Medical Association (JAMA)* called for more stringent regulations on dietary supplements, citing the potentially dangerous effects of ephedra.
- In early 2003, Napa County, California prosecutors sued Cytodyne Technologies, Inc., the maker of Xenadrine RFA-1 (the Steve Bechler supplement of choice), alleging the company has failed to disclose the link between the stimulant and health hazards, including myocardial infarction, strokes and death.
- Ephedra is prohibited by several professional and amateur sports-sanctioning bodies, including the NFL and the International Olympic Committee.
- On May 25, 2003, Illinois Governor Rod Blagojevich signed the nation's first statewide ban on ephedra, flanked by the parents of a sixteen-year-old football player who died of a heart attack after taking a product that contained ephedrine.

At first glance it's easy to believe ephedra is one troublesome herb and a public relations nightmare for the companies that sell it. That is, until you compare it to findings in various reports regarding over-the-counter and prescription drugs.

For instance, a study published in the *Journal of the American Medical Association* in 2000 showed that more than two million American hospital patients suffered a serious adverse drug reaction (ADR) within the twelve-month period of the study and, of these, over 100,000 died as a result. The researchers found that over 75 percent of these ADRs were dose-dependent, which suggests they were due to the inherent toxicity of the drugs rather than to allergic reactions. It's also important to note that the data did not include fatal reactions caused by accidental overdoses or errors in administration of the drugs. If these had been included, it is estimated that another 100,000 deaths would be added to the yearly total. The researchers concluded that ADRs *are now the fourth leading cause of death in the United States* after heart disease, cancer, and stroke.

Pretty scary numbers, yet the report elicited nothing like the outrage currently swirling around ephedra. (In fact, I'd be willing to bet big bucks that you've never heard of this risk associated with prescription drugs—am I right?)

It's Not Just Hospitals

Another recent study found that one in four patients who receive prescription drugs from primary care doctors experience harmful side effects. Some might say that I'm comparing apples and oranges. Prescription drugs are given to people who are already sick, and harmful side effects are the price they pay, whereas the use of ephedra for weight loss is not related to an illness per se, and its side effects are simply unnecessary and unacceptable.

While there is some merit in this line of thinking, I think it's instructive to look at this issue a little more closely. First, not all prescription drugs are necessary to cure illness. In fact, there is a considerable body of evidence showing that many drugs are prescribed for reasons other than necessity. These include pressure by the patient to prescribe a certain drug; lack of initiative on part of the patient and/or doctor to use proven lifestyle or non-drug therapies; use of drugs that merely relieve symptoms but do not "cure" the disease; and a failure to correctly identify the condition, which results in the prescribing of drugs that ultimately prove useless to the patient.

Let's look more closely at the aforementioned study about prescription drugs. According to the study, which appeared in the *New England Journal of Medicine,* the reactions resulting from prescriptions given by primary care physicians—such as rapid heart rate, sexual dysfunction, rash and nausea—are four times higher than those in patients who receive their medications in the hospital. The researchers said the findings are significant. Why? Because far more people receive their prescription drugs outside of a hospital, although most studies have focused on hospital-based reactions.

There are other relevant aspects to this topic. Poor communication between primary care doctors and patients contributed to the outpatient drug problems, with some allergies and drug interactions going unnoticed in rushed clinic visits, said the study's lead author, Dr. Tejal Gandhi of Brigham and Women's Hospital in Boston. "There are a lot of barriers to communication that you don't find in hospitals," Gandhi said. "If patients have to call the clinic, leave a message, wait for a call back and be asked to come in for a visit to report a problem, they may not."

Research methods also may explain why the new study found a higher rate of side effects. While most studies of drug reactions inside hospitals have relied on medical records, this study surveyed the patients themselves (661 to be exact) from four Boston doctors' offices. These patient surveys may have overcounted drug side effects, Dr. William Tierney of Indiana

University said in an editorial accompanying the study. Some patients attributed sexual dysfunction to drugs for depression, but depression often causes sexual problems, he said. "These symptoms are common among outpatients and may have nothing to do with their drug regimens," Tierney said. On the other hand, Gandhi said two doctors reviewed patient claims and ruled out many perceived side effects.

The study produced other intriguing, if not surprising, results:

- The drugs with the most problems were high blood pressure medications, nonsteroidal anti-inflammatory agents and selective serotonin-reuptake inhibitors, which are widely used to treat depression.
- Of the drug reactions, 13 percent were serious, and 39 percent could have been reduced or prevented.
- An elderly patient in the study who had a documented antibiotic allergy ended up in an emergency room for a body rash after being given the antibiotic.
- A middle-aged patient developed jaundice after taking a cholesterol-lowering drug and a pill for fungus, medications that shouldn't be administered together.

The researches claim there is much that can be done to prevent the high number of adverse reactions and errors in drug prescriptions. They noted that drug reactions could be curtailed through computerized drug ordering systems, e-mail between doctors and patients, patient-secure websites, nurse or pharmacist follow-up calls and education programs. Patients on multiple medications also should take a list of those drugs to every doctor appointment, they added.

The FDA says it is working with drug companies, the American Medical Association and consumer groups to seek ways to protect consumers. The FDA says one factor contributing to this dilemma is the pressure that patients and politicians

---

Side Effects, Prescription Errors and OTC Drugs

The problem of serious side effects caused by drugs is not just an American problem, and not only a problem with prescription drugs. In the U.K., it is estimated that over six hundred deaths a year are certified as being due to medicines sold over the counter, according to statistics compiled by the U.K.'s Office for National Statistics.

---

put on them for faster access to promising medications. The regulatory agency says in recent years it has moved drugs more rapidly through the regulatory pipeline, which, understandably, raises a drug's risk of increased or unknown side effects. In one recent two-year period, the FDA recalled five drugs and moved to re-evaluate several others, including the diabetes drug Rezulin.

Another factor behind the serious side effects or even death resulting from prescription drugs is that of people *not* following or understanding their dosing directions. Granted, a few may be so ill that it's hard for them to do so, but many just don't think it's that important and are nonchalant in their approach to using prescriptions. There's also the widespread mentality that if a little helps them, *a lot* will cure them even faster.

Ephedra and Weight Loss

So, what does all of this have to do with ephedra? Plenty, but before moving on, we need to look at the principal reason why ephedra products are used in this country. As I've mentioned, one of the main uses for ephedra today is to lose weight. And let's face it, if we look around (and perhaps into a mirror), many of us need to lose a few pounds. How bad is the problem?

According to the American Public Health Association (APHA), two-thirds of all American adults and nine million children between the ages of six and nineteen are overweight.

Approximately three hundred thousand deaths in the U.S. each year are directly related to obesity. The condition is associated with an increased risk of heart disease—the leading cause of death in the U.S.—as well as the currently surging rates of diabetes, certain cancers and other chronic ills.

A poll by APHA conducted in April 2003 showed that 63 percent of the six hundred American adults surveyed consider obesity to be a "major" public health threat, and 74 percent said they think the problem will keep getting worse.

"Lots of us are very much concerned about the effects of being overweight," said Dr. Georges Benjamin, executive director of the APHA. Benjamin said the issue that worries Americans the most is the alarming rate at which children are becoming obese. In fact, close to half of survey respondents said they were "very concerned" about kids being overweight. According to APHA, the proportion of children who are overweight has tripled since 1980. "Look on the streets and you just see it," says Dr. Benjamin. "There are just so many kids becoming overweight, and the numbers bear that out."

Although poor diet is an important factor in obesity, the poll results revealed that Americans place more emphasis on lack of exercise as a root problem.

One in four surveyed said the most important cause of adult obesity is a sedentary or "lazy" lifestyle, and a similar number said adults don't get enough exercise.

It's well understood that adolescence is a critical period for establishing lifetime weight management. The *American Journal of Clinical Nutrition* reports fully one-third of people who are overweight or obese as adults become that way during their first twenty years of life.

But even kids who aren't overweight are sensitive to media portrayals of what they should look like, and it's skinny. As a result, children as young as nine are going on diets after being taunted at school about being fat—even though many are normal weight for their age, psychologists from Leeds University in the U.K., reported in January 2003. They said dieting early in life can act as a trigger for eating disorders. Their study found 21 percent of girls and 16 percent of boys of primary school age were teased about being fat, causing loss of self-esteem. It's no wonder that opposite the binge and compulsive overeating side of the eating disorder spectrum we have the growing problem of anorexia nervosa and bulimia nervosa.

Enter Ephedra

As a society, we have learned to crave quick results as much as we do excess calories. We want to lose weight with little or no discomfort, and many of us want chiseled muscles quickly without the pain. When we compete in sports, we want that extra edge pushing us to the victory stand, and we're willing to get there by just about any means necessary. Rather than doing a few more crunches or push-ups or walking an extra mile, we opt for a medicated edge. In short, we want results with the lowest possible sacrifice.

Two crosscurrents are at work here. Our own internal fortitude and natural abilities versus our willingness—or unwillingness to be precise—to change our behavior. It's no wonder the weight loss industry, which includes ephedra sales, is a multibillion-dollar market.

But what if popular ephedra weight-loss products are taken off the market—will that cause people to seek other ways to lose weight, or will they simply resign themselves to a life of obesity? The market for ephedra has already been adversely affected. Several major manufacturers have discontinued their products, and numerous retailers have pulled ephedra products from their shelves due to safety concerns. In light of the death last February of Steve Bechler, Major League Baseball may soon join the National Football League in banning ephedrine or ephedra altogether.

Despite such risks, people are seeking a simple way to lose pounds fast, and will simply turn to other stimulants, says Katherine Beals, a nutrition professor at Ball State University. "Americans are looking for a quick fix," said Beals, a dedicated distance runner. "Rather than eating healthfully and exercising, which take time and effort, we would rather pop a pill to lose weight. A pill is thought to be infinitely easier and potentially quicker.

"Unfortunately, as we saw with fen-phen in the 1990s and now with ephedrine, it is also risky," she said. "Yet, a good many Americans are willing to take that risk and forsake their health in the name of looking good." Fen-phen became a dieting craze in the 1990s after research found a positive slimming effect from combining two appetite suppressants, fenfluramine and phentermine. Beals added that even the fallout caused by several deaths linked to ephedra products has hardly put a dent in the nation's hunger for weight-loss pills.

There's no doubt many of us need an attitude adjustment. But beyond that, why the differing levels of concern regarding problems with prescription drugs—which you rarely hear about—and ephedra, which generates bold headlines? Is it simply a question of not wanting the risks of an "unnecessary" medication, even though the chances of these risks are very small? Is that why we look the other way when the AMA reports numerous deaths from the popular non-steroidal anti-inflammatory drug (NSAIDs) ibuprofen, five hundred annual aspirin deaths or when the American Association of Poison Control Centers says more than one hundred people die from acetaminophen use? Is it because we believe all these medications are "safe" if taken as directed, and doctors and patients are completely aware of potential side effects?

If it's a question of safety versus benefit, why are we considering banning ephedra when we all know that tens of thousands of people die or are injured each year because of alcohol-related accidents, tens of thousands more suffer physical abuse at the hands of alcoholics, and cigarette smoking causes an average of 430,700 deaths a year? While both these substances have sale restrictions of sorts, you don't hear much noise about outright bans, do you? Could it be the way the "substances" are regulated and by whom?

Still, there are charges that the FDA is dragging its feet in banning ephedra because of the influence of powerful lobby groups and the amount of money at stake. This is probably the perfect time to examine and shed some light on the whole drug regulatory process.

CHAPTER 3

The FDA: Who's Regulating Whom?

THE FOOD AND DRUG ADMINISTRATION (FDA) touches the lives of every American every day. The FDA—which is part of the Department of Health and Human Services—regulates over $1 trillion worth of products, which is about one of every four dollars spent annually by American consumers. As impressive as this sounds, the FDA's reach is greater—and more controversial—than people realize. Consider this scenario:

You're at the doctor's office, and you've undergone a battery of tests. After sitting for some time on the examination table, the nurse pops in. Forcing a smile, she says after you remove the stiff paper gown you should meet with the doctor in his office.

On the way, you pass a well-groomed young man and woman hovering over a large spread of food. The doctor's staff surround the table, picking at the cold cuts, cheeses and an assortment of cookies and fruit. You have a chance to look around the doctor's office before he comes in. You see his degrees and stacks of files, printouts and large manila envelopes labeled "radiology."

The doctor sits down behind his desk. He looks grim. He tells you both your blood pressure and cholesterol count are too high, and if you don't lose weight you're a prime candidate for diabetes. For these he scribbles out two prescriptions. He then says that your heartburn complaints are due to gastroesophageal reflux disease, known as GERD, which also could be caused by the extra pounds you're carrying. He recommends you take Prilosec.

He starts to write a prescription for it and stops. He tells you it's unnecessary since Prilosec is now available over-the-counter. Almost as an afterthought he slides two vacuum-sealed plastic packets towards you. "In the meantime, why don't you take these?"

On the way out, you notice that the sparkling well-heeled man and woman by the food spread have nametags. You realize they're sales reps for a major pharmaceutical company.

At the drugstore, the pharmacist tells you they have a generic equivalent for only one of your prescriptions. You cringe, knowing your health plan requires a higher co-pay for brand-name medicine.

As you wait for the prescriptions to be filled, you grab the Prilosec and head for the vitamin shelves. As you browse, you look at the label of one popular brand and see it contains over 500 percent more of one vitamin than is recommended. You put it back, fearing an overdose.

The next few rows contain a wide variety and assortment of vitamins, minerals, herbs and other supplements, including ginseng, garlic, coQ10—whatever that might be—vitamin E, a B-complex vitamin, trimethylglycine (which you can't even pronounce) and licorice root. You chuckle to yourself when you see bottles of fish oil, green tea extract and grape seed extract. "What a waste of money," you think to yourself. You eat plenty—maybe too much—but you're sure you get all the nutrients you need. Why eat grapes or fish in a pill? Probably just expensive urine, you figure.

Then you begin looking over the diet pills. One catches your eye—it has a picture of a man with washboard abs. You check the ingredients to make sure it doesn't contain ephedra, since you've read it kills people. An ingredient you don't recognize, synephrine, is listed. The label describes it as an "effective and safe ephedra substitute." You shrug and put it in your basket, not really knowing whether or not its ingredients are effective—or safe, for that matter.

Pretty soon, you've drifted over to the food section. You brighten when you see a box of "artificial sweetener" near the low-fat potato chips. You figure you can reduce calories by using aspartame instead of sugar.

Your prescription is still not ready, so you sit in the waiting area and watch the overhead TV. During a break there are three drug commercials: one for an allergy medicine, another for acid reflux disease, and one for impotence. You blush, and head back to the prescription counter. The pharmacist rummages through dozens of white bags with forms stapled to the front. He soon hands you two bags. As you head for the register, you pass the shelves of pain relievers. Remembering that you're out of Tylenol, you grab a bottle.

What does this little scenario have to do with the FDA and ephedra? More importantly, what does it have to do with you? As you'll see, plenty.

Everything You Ever Wanted to Know About the FDA

It should come as no surprise to anyone who follows today's health news that numerous studies have validated many of the health claims for vitamins, minerals and herbs the FDA had earlier rejected (some say suppressed). For example, the FDA for years refused to acknowledge research data concerning vitamin E and heart health. Since ephedra is an herb, the FDA considers it neither a food nor a drug, and thus is regulated as a dietary supplement—an entirely different category with its own set of rules. This is probably a good place to back up a little.

The FDA is one of our nation's oldest consumer-protection agencies. Its nine thousand employees monitor the manufacture, import, transport, storage and sale of about $1 trillion worth of products each year, costing taxpayers about $3 per person.

First and foremost, the FDA is a public health agency, charged with protecting American consumers by enforcing the Federal Food, Drug, and Cosmetic Act (FD&C Act) and several related public health laws. To do this, the FDA has some 1,100 investigators and inspectors in district and local offices in 157 cities across the country, covering nearly 95,000 FDA-regulated businesses.

The FDA originated in the late 1930s after the Massengil company marketed an antibiotic product called Elixir Sulfanilamide without prior toxicity testing of its solvent. The solvent—diethylene glycol (which is used today as automotive antifreeze)—caused the death of 107 people, mostly children. The "Elixir Sulfanilamide tragedy" prompted the passage of the FD&C Act in 1938 and eventually led to the establishment of the FDA.

Today the FD&C Act authorizes the FDA to regulate drugs, medical devices, foods and cosmetics under different standards. For decades, the FDA regulated dietary supplements as foods, in most circumstances, to ensure that they were safe and wholesome, and that their labeling was truthful and not misleading. An important facet of ensuring safety was the FDA's power to judge the safety of all new ingredients, including those used in dietary supplements, granted to it by the 1958 Food Additive Amendments to the FD&C Act.

Other FDA Tasks

Another major FDA mission is to protect the safety and

wholesomeness of food. The agency's scientists test samples to see if any substances, such as pesticide residues, are present in unacceptable amounts. If contaminants are identified, the FDA takes corrective action. The FDA also sets labeling standards to help consumers know what is in the foods they buy. Another FDA responsibility is to make sure medicated feeds and other drugs given to animals raised for food do not threaten the health of consumers.

The FDA is also responsible for the safety of the nation's blood supply. The agency's investigators routinely examine blood bank operations, from record-keeping to testing for contaminants. The FDA also ensures the purity and effectiveness of biologicals (medical preparations made from living organisms and their products), such as insulin and vaccines.

Medical devices are classified and regulated according to their degree of risk to the public. Devices that are life-supporting, life-sustaining or implanted, such as pacemakers, must receive agency approval before they can be marketed. After a drug or device is approved for marketing, the agency collects and analyzes tens of thousands of reports each year to monitor for any unexpected adverse reactions.

Cosmetic safety also comes under the FDA's jurisdiction. The agency can remove unsafe cosmetics from the marketplace. The dyes, preservatives and other additives used in drugs, foods and cosmetics must pass FDA scrutiny and the agency must review and approve these chemicals before they can be used.

Unlike most drugs and devices, foods (and dietary supplements) do not require pre-market approval because of their inherent safety and history of use. Rather, the law requires that manufacturers of dietary supplements, prior to marketing, submit data to the FDA for any new dietary ingredient that is not already present in the food supply.

If a company is found violating any of the laws that the FDA enforces, the agency can "persuade" the firm to voluntarily correct the problem or to recall a faulty product from the market.

A recall is generally the fastest and most effective way to protect the public from an unsafe product.

When a company can't (or won't) voluntarily correct a public health problem with one of its products, the FDA can bring to bear legal sanctions. The agency can go to court to force a company to stop selling a product and to have items already produced seized and destroyed. When warranted, criminal penalties—including prison sentences—are sought against manufacturers and distributors.

About three thousand products a year are found to be unfit for consumers and are withdrawn from the marketplace, either by voluntary recall or by court-ordered seizure. In addition, about thirty thousand import shipments a year are detained at port of entry because the goods appear to be unacceptable.

Should Vitamins, Minerals and Herbs Be Classified as Drugs?

For decades the FDA tried to regulate the sale and use of vitamins, herbs, and other dietary supplements. By law, the FDA ruled that any ingested product intended by its manufacturer to prevent or treat a disease is a drug. Products (other than "food") that are intended to affect the structure or function of the body are also considered drugs. Throughout the 1950s and 1960s, the FDA brought hundreds of court actions against nutrition manufacturers for making health-related claims for their products. Under threat of law, food manufacturers were even prevented from labeling the fat, cholesterol, or other nutritional content of their food. (*Note:* Such labeling was later allowed, and with the Nutrition Labeling and Education Act of 1990, nutrition labeling became mandatory.)

The FDA actively prosecuted vitamin retailers that sold vitamins and other supplements in conjunction with books or pamphlets that extolled their use. It was illegal for a health food store to sell vitamins and books touting the virtues of vitamins.

The FDA justified such practices, which many considered to be a violation of the First Amendment, under the theory that literature sold near a product was thereby converted into a product label, and if health claims were made in the literature, then the product had to be regulated as a drug (and thus had to go through FDA clinical trials before being sold).

In 1973, the FDA published regulations expanding its control over supplements by declaring that any dietary supplement that it considered to lack nutritional usefulness was a drug and thus under the FDA's control. The regulations took effect in 1975. For instance, high-potency vitamins, defined by the FDA as vitamins sold in dosages as little as twice the federal recommended daily allowance (RDA), were automatically considered drugs.

As a result, high-potency vitamins were effectively made illegal by this ruling because they could not be sold without FDA approval, and the FDA would not approve supplements that it considered to be "unnecessary." Vitamin manufacturers and consumers fought back, and in response Congress passed the Proxmire Vitamin Mineral Amendment of 1976, which stated that the FDA could not classify a mineral or vitamin as a drug "solely because it exceeds the level of potency the FDA determines is nutritionally rational or useful."

Under the protection of the Proxmire Amendment, the dietary and nutritional supplement industry expanded. Undaunted, the FDA stepped up enforcement again in the early 1990s after thirty-eight deaths were attributed to L-tryptophan, an amino acid widely used for treating depression and building muscle mass. (*Note:* The Centers for Disease Control later exonerated L-tryptophan in the deaths, which were caused by a contaminant and not L-tryptophan. However, the FDA did not lift its ban on over-the-counter sales of L-tryptophan.)

In 1985, the FDA lost a bitter turf battle with the Federal Trade Commission (FTC) and the National Institutes of Health (NIH). Under recommendation from the National Cancer

Institute, a division of the NIH, the FTC permitted Kellogg's to claim that a high-fiber diet reduced the probability of certain types of cancer. The FDA wanted to sue Kellogg, but the FTC argued that the ads presented "important public health recommendations in an accurate, useful, and substantiated way." Under pressure, the FDA backed down, and as a result it was established that food products could advertise a "substantiated" health claim without going through the FDA drug approval process. Later, in 1993, the FDA announced that it planned to regulate as drugs all amino acids, herbs, and other supplements including fibers and fish oils. The FDA immediately found itself under a furious attack from millions of consumers and the supplement industry in general.

Enter DSHEA

In response to the rising controversy between the FDA and its regulation of the supplement industry, the Dietary Supplement Health and Education Act (DSHEA) was passed in 1994. With passage of the DSHEA, Congress amended the FD&C Act to include several provisions that apply only to dietary supplements and ingredients of dietary supplements. As a result, this new law created a new regulatory framework for the safety and labeling of dietary supplements.

Signed by President Clinton on October 25, 1994, the DSHEA acknowledges that millions of consumers believe dietary supplements may help augment daily diets and provide health benefits. Congress' intent in enacting the DSHEA was to meet the concerns of consumers and manufacturers and to help ensure that safe and appropriately labeled products remain available for those who want to use them.

In the findings associated with the DSHEA, Congress stated that there may be a positive relationship between sound dietary practice and good health, and that, although further scientific research is needed, there may be a connection between dietary supplement use, reduced health-care expenses, and disease prevention.

So, what allowances do the DSHEA codes make for supplement manufacturers and distributors? Under the DSHEA, nutritional supplements can make substantiated "statements of nutritional support" that do not thereby invoke FDA control. Supplements, however, cannot make claims regarding disease without becoming regulated as drugs. The distinction between statements of nutritional support and claims regarding disease is vague. Manufacturers of St. John's wort, for example, may claim that St. John's wort "promotes healthy emotional balance and well-being," but they cannot say St. John's wort "is useful in the treatment of depression." The difference is of most interest to lawyers—not consumers—when you consider how many people take St. John's wort for mild cases of depression (more on this later).

Under DSHEA, a supplement company is responsible for determining that the product it manufactures or distributes is safe and that any representations or claims made about it are not false or misleading and are supported by adequate evidence. This means that dietary supplements do not need approval from the FDA before they are marketed. Except in the case of a new dietary ingredient, where pre-market review for safety data and other information is required, a manufacturer does not have to provide the FDA with the evidence it relies on to substantiate safety or effectiveness before or after it begins to market its products. The thinking is that these ingredients have already passed muster for safety.

As a result of these provisions, dietary ingredients used in supplements are not subject to the pre-market safety evaluations required of other new food ingredients or for new uses of old food ingredients. They must, however, meet the requirements of other safety provisions.

The FDA Modernization Act of 1997

By the late 1990s, numerous academic studies and government reports had indicted the FDA for "dragging its feet" regarding the approval of drugs and the monitoring of them afterwards. Pressure for reform finally began to be felt by members of Congress, a portion of which had recently promised deregulation in their "Contract with America." In 1996, the House wrote an FDA reform bill that would have significantly threatened some of the FDA's central powers, but the FDA and its supporters in the Clinton administration defeated it. Facing a veto, Congress abandoned the bill and the following year passed a watered-down bill, the FDA Modernization Act of 1997.

Much of the Modernization Act merely put in writing what was already FDA practice. For one thing, it authorizes the FDA to appoint panels of scientific experts to assist the agency in evaluating new drugs, a practice the FDA has followed for decades. Similarly, it codified the rule that only one adequate and well-controlled clinical study in addition to confirmatory evidence could be the basis of approval for a new drug. The most important provisions of this act were the reauthorization of user fees for another five years. As you'll see later in this chapter, these user fees are very controversial.

The FDA's Powers

A dietary supplement that is adulterated or misbranded or bears an unauthorized drug claim can be seized, condemned and destroyed. A perfect illustration of this ability occurred recently when the Federal Trade Commission and FDA charged the marketers of a dietary supplement called Coral Calcium Supreme with making false and unsubstantiated claims about the product's health benefits, especially during their oft-seen

Drugs and Dietary Supplements: What Are the Differences?

Stated as simply as possible:
· Drugs treat, cure, diagnose or prevent abnormal states.
· Dietary supplements maintain normal, healthy states.

Under DSHEA, a dietary supplement is "a natural substance which goes beyond essential nutrients to include other substances such as ginseng, garlic, fish oils, psyllium, enzymes, glandulars, and mixtures of these." According to DSHEA, a dietary supplement is:

· A product, other than tobacco, which is used in conjunction with a healthy diet and contains one or more of the following dietary ingredients: a vitamin, mineral, herb or other botanical, an amino acid, a dietary substance for use by man to supplement the diet by increasing the total daily intake, or a concentrate, metabolite, constituent, extract, or combinations of these ingredients.
· Intended for ingestion in pill, capsule, tablet or liquid form.
· Not represented for use as a conventional food or as the sole item of a meal or diet.
· Labeled as a "dietary supplement."

This includes products such as an approved new drug, certified antibiotic, or licensed biologic that was marketed as a dietary supplement or food before approval, certification, or license (unless the Secretary of Health and Human Services waives this provision).

infomercials on cable TV. In a complaint filed in federal district court, the agencies allege that Kevin Trudeau, Robert Barefoot, Shop America (USA), LLC and Deonna Enterprises, Inc. violated the FTC Act by claiming, falsely and without substantiation, that Coral Calcium Supreme can treat or cure cancer and other diseases such as multiple sclerosis and heart disease.

The DSHEA codes include other safety requirements regarding the introduction of new dietary ingredients. The law clarified that dietary supplement ingredients marketed prior to October 15, 1994 do not require pre-market approval. However, manufacturers marketing a new dietary supplement ingredient after this date must submit safety information on the new dietary ingredient to the FDA.

The FDA can remove products from the market for the following reasons:

- *The Product Poses a Significant and Unreasonable Risk*: The FDA does not have to prove that a product actually harmed anyone, but simply that it presents a "significant or unreasonable risk" of illness or injury.
- *The Product Contains Poisonous or Deleterious Substances*: The FDA does not have to prove that a product has a substance that will injure, but simply that it *may* render injury under the recommended or suggested conditions indicated on a product's label.
- *The Product Is Unfit for Food*: The FDA has authority to stop the marketing of any dietary supplement that the agency believes is not fit for human consumption.
- *The Product Makes Drug Claims*: If a dietary supplement's label indicates that the product can diagnose, cure, mitigate, treat or prevent a disease, then it is clearly being represented as a "drug" and is no longer considered a dietary supplement. Responsible manufacturers have labels, warnings, and directions for use for their products and are careful not to represent their products as drugs. As in the coral calcium case I mentioned above, the FTC and FDA charges that these and other claims go far beyond existing scientific evidence regarding the recognized health benefits of calcium. This action, by the way, is part of a series of initiatives the FTC and the FDA are taking against the purveyors of products with unsubstantiated health and medical claims.

- *The Product Lacks Truthful and Informative Labeling:* By law, all dietary supplement products must contain extensive informative labeling, including detailed information about the nutrients in the product, such as name and quantity of all ingredients in the product and the name and place of business of the company. (By the way, most legitimate companies in the dietary supplement industry support the enforcement of this provision.)

Recently the Secretary of Health and Human Services announced enforcement efforts to remove products that were marketed to minors and for illicit purposes. The supplement industry has consistently urged the FDA to use its enforcement powers to remove such products from the marketplace.

DSHEA also provides the Secretary of Health and Human Services with the authority to remove *any* dietary supplement or supplement ingredient that poses an "imminent hazard." If the HHS Secretary makes this decision, the government must conduct an administrative review of the case and the product cannot be sold to the public.

Familiar Words

Dietary supplements that make nutritional claims must carry the following two disclaimers which are probably familiar to most of us:

- "This statement has not been evaluated by the Food and Drug Administration."
- "This product is not intended to diagnose, treat, cure, or prevent any disease."

Though subject to certain conditions, such as that the information presented is not false or misleading and not biased in favor of a particular manufacturer or brand, DSHEA also restricts the FDA's ability to ban the dissemination of information on dietary supplements. Health food retailers, for example, can now market books, magazines, and scientific literature describing the uses of dietary supplements. As a result, in recent years consumers have had much more information—for better or worse, some may argue—pertaining to the health benefits of vitamins and other supplements.

Ephedra Comes on the Scene

Due to pressure from numerous negative press stories—including the death of Steve Bechler—in February 2003 the Department of Health and Human Services announced a number of actions to address concerns about ephedra's safety. First, warning letters were sent to dozens of ephedra manufacturers, challenging them to remove unproven claims or substantiate those claims, with a particular focus on athletic performance enhancement claims.

HHS stated that given what they see as limited evidence of ephedra's benefits, the FDA and the Federal Trade Commission are assessing whether further enforcement actions are warranted against other manufacturers. Meanwhile, a new, mandatory warning label for all ephedra products was proposed. It would make it clear to users, via a black-box warning on the front of the product, as well as additional information in the product labeling, that "serious adverse events and death have been reported after using ephedra, and that risks of adverse events are particularly high with strenuous exercise and/or use of stimulants, including caffeine."

Additionally, the FDA announced it was seeking comments from health professionals, the supplement industry, and the general public on any additional data regarding ephedra's safety, with the promise of compiling an accurate image of ephedra's potential risks.

More on this, and how the FDA's powers affect ephedra, will follow in a later chapter.

Different Standards

Prescription drugs need to undergo various steps before they are approved for use (see the sidebar "How a Drug is Approved"). The industry boldly claims the cost of developing a new prescription drug is probably over $800 million. The consumer watchdog group Public Citizen scoffs at this estimate. Suspecting the pharmaceutical industry is either not being truthful or they have really lousy accountants, they believe the true figure is more than likely at least 75 percent lower; in large part because much of the research is conducted under government grants.

One thing is for sure—drug companies aren't too fond of untested dietary supplements that compete against their drugs. Especially when you consider that supplements can bypass the costly FDA approval process by simply carrying a statement saying the product hasn't been evaluated by the FDA.

The FDA, Controversy, and Conflicts of Interest

According to *USA Today,* in October 2000 the well-known pharmaceutical company Johnson & Johnson sent a team of executives to a Holiday Inn ballroom in Silver Spring, Maryland for a specific purpose—to persuade the FDA's panel of independent experts that an expensive antibiotic, Levaquin, should be the first drug approved to treat penicillin-resistant pneumonia.

For Johnson & Johnson executives, the FDA's Anti-Infective Drug Advisory Committee included some people it knew quite well. At least two of the experts were paid consultants to the

How a Drug Is Approved

Drug companies study thousands of compounds before settling on the very few that might eventually prove to have therapeutic value. During the six to seven years of preclinical testing (including animal testing), of five thousand compounds tested, approximately five will show enough promise for a company to file an Investigational New Drug Application (IND). If the IND is approved by the FDA and by an Institutional Review Board, the manufacturer can begin the first phase of development.

The IND stage consists of three phases:

Phase I: Clinical trials using healthy individuals are conducted to determine the drug's basic properties and safety profile in humans. Typically the drug remains in this stage for one to two years.

Phase II: Efficacy trials begin as the drug is administered to volunteers of the target population. At the end of phase II, the manufacturer meets with FDA officials to discuss the development process, continued human testing, any questions the FDA has, and the protocols for phase III.

Phase III: This is usually the most extensive and most expensive part of drug development, including additional human clinical trials.

(*Note:* During the phases of the IND, the manufacturer can obtain accelerated development/review of the drug.)

Once phase III is complete, the manufacturer files a New Drug Application (NDA.) Review of the NDA typically lasts one to two years, bringing total drug development and approval (that is, the IND and NDA stages) to approximately nine years. During the NDA stage, the FDA consults advisory committees made of experts to obtain a broader range of advice on drug safety, effectiveness, and labeling. Once approved, the drug may be marketed with FDA regulated labeling.

The FDA also gathers safety information as the drug is used and adverse events are reported, and will occasionally request changes in labeling or will submit press releases as new contraindications arise. If adverse events appear to be systematic and serious, the FDA may withdraw a product from the market.

drug company and had worked on the very same medicine they were being asked to evaluate for approval in an important new market.

The expert panel's "consumer representative," whose assignment is to defend consumers' interests, had the most extensive financial relationship with Johnson & Johnson. Keith Rodvold, a pharmacy professor at the University of Illinois-Chicago, served on a company anti-infective drug advisory board, according to Johnson & Johnson spokesman Marc Monseau. Rodvold advised the company on how to design and analyze the clinical trials that got the drug approved. In 1999, he designed a study to measure how Levaquin is absorbed in the lungs. The company also used him regularly as a consultant on a variety of issues.

When approached by *USA Today,* Rodvold declined to discuss his relationship with Johnson & Johnson and his work on Levaquin. Likewise, J&J would not say how much Rodvold had been paid during the five years of consulting with the company.

The case of Levaquin shows how deeply money and influence from the pharmaceutical industry can penetrate the drug approval process. The fact is, FDA advisory committees consist almost entirely of pharmaceutical industry consultants and researchers. Even consumers' and patients' representatives on the committees—the folks who are supposed to look out for you and me—often receive drug company money.

The law requires the FDA to screen all committee members for financial conflicts. It states members have conflicts when committee action could have the "direct and predictable effect" of causing the member a financial gain or loss. The only way around it is for the agency to issue a waiver, usually on the grounds that the experts' value outweighs the seriousness of the conflict. The FDA grants these waivers routinely.

In the period analyzed by *USA Today,* the FDA granted 803 conflict-of-interest waivers. In seventy-one other instances, members had financial conflicts that were voluntarily disclosed but did not require a waiver. In the 746 other member appearances on the committees, there was no conflict of interest.

Dallying for Dollars

While the FDA is required to disclose the existence of financial conflicts, it has kept details under wraps since 1992, making it nearly impossible to uncover the amount of money or the drug company involved. Since then, the FDA stopped making public the details of financial conflicts after controversies about whether the financial interests of committee members had unduly influenced decisions on breast implants, Prozac and a drug to treat Alzheimer's disease. The FDA said it stopped releasing details on conflicts because of concerns about violating the privacy rights of committee members—not because of the controversies.

In its research, *USA Today* found at least one committee member had a financial stake in the topic under review at 146 of 159 FDA advisory committee meetings held from January 1, 1998, through June 30, 2000. At eighty-eight of those meetings, at least half the advisory committee members had financial interests in the topic being evaluated; at 92 percent of the meetings, at least one member had a financial conflict of interest; at the 102 meetings dealing with the fate of a specific drug, 33 percent of the experts had a financial conflict. As you would expect, more often than not the FDA followed the committees' advice.

After the *USA Today* story broke, FDA senior associate commissioner Linda Suydam, who was in charge of waiving conflict-of-interest restrictions, defended the FDA's practices. "The best experts for the FDA are often the best experts to consult with industry," she said.

The experts hired to advise the FDA assist in deciding which medicines should be approved for sale, what the warning labels should say and how studies of drugs should be designed. It might seem unnecessary for the FDA to seek outside advice. After all, the agency employs its own full complement of scientific specialists. But the FDA says outside experts add a wide spectrum of judgment, outlook, and state-of-the-art experience to drug issues confronting the FDA. "We seek scientists with a broad range of expertise and different backgrounds," said John Treacy, director of the advisors and consultants staff in the FDA's Center for Drug Evaluation and Research (CDER).

The FDA believes expert advisers add to the agency's understanding, so that final agency decisions will more likely reflect a balanced evaluation. While committee recommendations are not binding, the agency considers them carefully when deciding drug issues.

The FDA said most members of its drug advisory committees are physicians whose specialties involve the drugs under the purview of their committee. Others include registered nurses, statisticians, epidemiologists and pharmacologists (who study drug effects in the body). Consumer-nominated members serve on all committees. As voting members, they must possess scientific expertise to participate fully in deliberations. They must have worked with consumer groups so they can assess the impact of decisions on consumers.

This does not jive with what *USA Today* found. The paper discovered that more than half of the experts hired to advise the government on the safety and effectiveness of medicine have financial relationships with the pharmaceutical companies that had a financial stake in the decisions. In other words, very often the people playing critical roles in making decisions affecting the health and well-being of millions of Americans and influencing billions of dollars in drugs sales are people who benefit financially.

"The industry has more influence on the process than people realize," said Larry Sasich, a pharmacist who works for Public Citizen's Health Research Group, a consumer advocacy organization founded by Ralph Nader. "It is outrageous that the pharmaceutical industry's influence is so great that even some consumer representatives are on drug companies' payrolls."

Another Big "Uh-Oh!"

Because of the increased expense due to reforms and other costs, the FDA, Congress and the pharmaceutical industry negotiated the Prescription Drug User Fee Act of 1992. In essence, these user fees "forced" (or allowed, depending on your take) drug companies to pay a portion of the FDA' s cost to review marketing applications for drugs.

Since user fees were first authorized ten years ago, the FDA has taken in $162 million dollars from the pharmaceutical industry. User fees also have provided Congress with a good reason to continue to underfund the FDA. As a result, the agency often cannot carry out many of the public protection duties assigned to it.

Since the inception of the user fees, the FDA's staff devoted exclusively to new drug and biologics pre-approval has doubled—financed in part by the user fees—while staff for all other oversight activities has shrunk by 15 percent. As a result, there aren't enough inspectors to regularly visit drug manufacturing plants in the U.S. and abroad to make sure good manufacturing standards are maintained, nor are there enough to regularly inspect the safety of the thousands of food products that come under FDA authority. Before the introduction of user fees, the FDA was free to allocate its resources as its scientists felt necessary. Now, a smaller discretionary budget means some important items do not receive funding.

Back to Our Scenario

As you can see, the FDA wields enormous clout over what we eat, drink and take as "medicine." Because of this power there are plenty of outside factors trying to muscle in and influence their regulatory authority and decisions. Remember the scenario we set up at the beginning of the chapter? Let's go back and examine other ways in which our well-being is often compromised.

On the way to the doctor's office, we passed a young man and woman hovering over a food table. We later learn that they're pharmaceutical sales representatives. There are currently approximately eighty thousand pharmaceutical sales people in the United States, which is slightly more than one for each ten physicians. The cost of face-to-face promotion (or detailing) in 2000 was approximately $4.8 billion, or *$6,400 for each practicing physician* in the United States. It's quite obvious that these reps are exerting significant influence over physicians.

According to industry estimates, drug companies spent $15.7 billion dollars on promotion in 2000. Over $7 billion worth of free samples were distributed that year. According to a study from the Department of Medicine at the University of Washington, pharmaceutical companies often use drug samples as a marketing strategy. Based on interviews with 131 doctors, they found the availability of drug samples led physicians to dispense and subsequently prescribe drugs that differ from their preferred drug choice. While physicians most often report using

The University of Washington Study

Here are a few more details about the study from the University of Washington. The researchers asked physicians to self-report their pre-scribing patterns for three clinical scenarios, including their preferred drug choice, whether they would use a drug sample and subsequently prescribe the sampled medication, and the importance of factors involved in the decision to dispense a drug sample. A total of 131 (85 percent) of 154 physicians responded. When presented with an insured woman with an uncomplicated lower urinary tract infection, 22 (17 percent) respondents reported that they would dispense a drug sample; 21 (95 percent) of these sample users stated that they would dispense a drug sample that differed from their preferred drug choice. For an uninsured man with hypertension, 35 (27 percent) respondents reported that they would dispense a drug sample; 32 (91 percent) of 35 sample users indicated that they would dispense a drug sample instead of their preferred drug choice. For an uninsured woman with depression, 108 (82 percent) respondents reported that they would dispense a drug sample; 53 (49 percent) of 108 sample users indicated that avoiding cost to the patient was the most consistent motivator for dispensing a drug sample for all three scenarios.

drug samples to avoid cost to the patient, they would dispense a drug sample that differed from their preferred drug choice.

What does this mean? While your physician undoubtedly had to go through a grueling medical school curriculum after college, many pharmaceutical sales reps have only a bachelor's degree and/or marketing background. This wouldn't much matter except when you consider the major pull that pharmaceutical sales reps have over what ends up in your medicine cabinet.

On the Other Hand

Not everyone agrees with the notion that pharmaceutical reps have too much power and influence. One recent study suggests that doctors are more wary of pharmaceutical companies' aggressive marketing than generally believed and don't easily yield to pressure to switch prescriptions. In a study presented at a conference of the Institute for Operations Research and the Management Sciences at the Robert H. Smith School of Business in the University of Maryland in June 2003, Natalie Mizik of Columbia University and Robert Jacobson of the University of Washington write, "Are physicians easy marks? To the contrary, our results show that physicians are 'tough sells' in that sales force activity has modest to very small influence on prescribing behavior."

The authors, noting accusations that pharmaceutical sales representatives (PSRs) compromise physician integrity, obtained access to a database that allowed them to assess the impact that interactions with sales reps have on the number of new prescriptions issued by physicians.

The study sample involved three different drugs and 74,075 American physicians. The database contained information for twenty-four months on the number of new prescriptions issued for a drug by a given physician, the number of "detailing" sales calls the physician received that month for the drug, and the number of free drug samples that the rep left with a physician. The data was provided on condition of anonymity.

The drugs differ: they come from different therapeutic areas; they have been on the market from less than one year to eleven years; and they have achieved different levels of commercial success—their annual sales range from under $500 million to over $1 billion. In total, the data represent over four million interactions between physicians and pharmaceutical sales representatives.

For each of the drugs in the study the authors used statistical modeling and operations research methods to assess the effect of changes in the amount of detailing and sampling on the number of additional new prescriptions the physician issued over the subsequent six-month period for the drug.

They found that pharmaceutical companies had to invest heavily to produce even a small increase in prescriptions. For the three drugs studied—drug 1 is prescribed by psychologists and psychiatrists, drugs 2 and 3 are prescribed by primary care physicians—the results indicate that it would take an additional 0.64, 3.11 and 6.54 visits by pharmaceutical sales reps, respectively, to induce one additional new prescription and 6.44, 25.39, and 73.05 additional free drug samples to induce one new prescription.

The authors say that the most important reason why sales reps are having limited influence is that they are not the only source of information for physicians. Doctors consult scientific papers, advice from colleagues, and their own experience when developing prescribing practices. "Indeed, most physicians view these influences as far more important than that of PSRs," write the authors. "Many physicians view skeptically or hold negative attitudes toward PSRs. They recognize that information presented is biased toward the promoted drug and is unlikely to be objective."

Benefit of Drug Samples

A related study by a second set of researchers at the same conference suggests that distributing drug samples is less a method to sway physicians than a way of contrasting medications and helping manufacturers maintain market share.

In "Prescription Drug Promotion: The Role and Value of Physicians' Samples Under Competition," Kissan Joseph of the University of Kansas and Murali K. Mantrala of ZS Associates in Evanston, Illinois, used a math model to analyze drug samples' impact on patients, physicians, and pharmaceutical manufacturers. They conclude that supplying samples plays a positive role in making the choice between medications.

"While critics often argue that this practice adversely affects patient welfare," they write, "we contend that samples provide a benefit by facilitating the match between drugs and patients' underlying disease state by reducing the cost of comparing drugs."

If patients are incorrectly matched to a drug, the researchers observe, they lose money and suffer the lack of physical relief from their ailment. Providing free samples helps reduce out-of-pocket cost to patients and alleviates some of the non-financial costs as well.

Surprisingly, they suggest that pharmaceutical companies are often the losers in the samples war, incurring great expense by distributing free samples purely as a defensive marketing tactic to maintain market share. Still, while this might sound logical, I believe that we should expect doctors and healthcare professionals to make their medical decisions based on science, not marketing.

Hypothetical Health Risks

While we're on the subject of prescriptions, it's important to note a few other things in the illustrative situation at the pharmacy. Remember all the prescription bags on the pharmacist's table? Granted, doctors in the U.S. write three billion prescriptions each year, yet according to the Institute of Medicine, prescription errors due to misreading physician's handwriting kill up to seven thousand Americans annually. In addition, overmedication and adverse reactions to prescription drugs also cause unnecessary deaths. In 1994, these accounted for 106,000 deaths, according to the *Journal of the American Medical Association*. In fact, more people are killed by adverse reactions to prescription drugs than by pulmonary disease or accidents. To top it off, it's now estimated an average of 137,000 people die each year just as a result of taking prescription medication where no mistakes or abuse is involved. Today, prescription drug deaths are surpassed only by heart disease, cancer, and stroke. The elderly, whose bodies often can't tolerate the dosages and combinations of pills doctors prescribe them, are particularly susceptible.

We also have to consider that while many drug interactions may not kill people, they do seriously injure them. Studies estimate that two million Americans are hospitalized annually from drug side effects. True, some dangerous drug side effects are simply a consequence of taking medicine, such as when chemotherapy treatments leave a patient vulnerable to infection.

There's another aspect of this problem. New drugs are tested on only a few hundred to a few thousand patients before they're sold to millions, meaning rare side effects that didn't show up in clinical studies can wind up hurting hundreds of people.

Part of the FDA's job is to track side effects of the medication after it's approved for sale so that health officials can take action if unexpected problems arise, and to develop strategies for preventing drug-related injuries. But the FDA learned of just 9,961 medication-related deaths and 33,541 hospitalizations in 1997, said a 1998 report from the Health and Human Services inspector general. Why? The problem lies in the voluntary nature of the injury reporting system, the report said. In simple terms, the FDA can require drug manufacturers to report only the injuries they learn about that involve their drugs. The FDA does not have the authority to require doctors and hospitals to report injuries, either to the government or to the drug companies themselves. But unless the FDA finds proactive ways to uncover patterns of injuries, it can't take the next step of helping to prevent them, the inspector general concluded.

Here's a perfect illustration. At the first World Congress on Lung Health and Respiratory Diseases in Florence, Italy, where fifteen thousand specialists from eighty-four countries met in September 2002, researchers noted there are hundreds of medicines routinely prescribed against a variety of disorders, including high blood pressure, allergies, rheumatism, certain cancers or even common non-respiratory inflammations that can cause all kinds of lung diseases. These diseases can develop within a very short time or after several years. They are mostly unpredictable and some are irreversible, resulting in permanent damage. Yet the information provided with the packaging rarely warns patients that the medicine could potentially cause a lung disorder, and there still aren't many doctors who even know to give the matter due thought when they prescribe a treatment.

Bet you never heard about this, right? It's somewhat ironic when you read in the press a negative article on supplements—they always talk about the lack of government regulation, which must mean that the safety of these products is highly questionable. Yet by comparison, nutritional supplements void of government regulation seem to be far more safe than highly regulated and enormously profitable prescription drugs.

Consider this—remember our patient looking over the wide selection of assorted vitamins? While there have been over 500 studies published in the medical literature about the dangers of homocysteine, our patient had never heard about it—not even from his doctor. While our patient of course knew about cholesterol (although he could never keep straight whether HDL was the good one or the bad one), elevations in homocysteine can lead to arteriosclerosis of the blood vessels in the heart and brain and is up to five times more deadly than elevated cholesterol. It is widely accepted that vitamins B6, B12, folic acid and trimethylglycine promote healthy homocysteine levels.

As for the patient's heartburn, licorice increases the production of protective mucus in the stomach and may reduce acid secretion, making it a useful treatment of inflammatory stomach conditions. It contains vitamin E, B-complex vitamins, biotin, niacin, pantothenic acid, lecithin, manganese and other trace elements. One warning for our patient, though—it shouldn't be used by people with hypertension.

As for Prilosec, the drug the doctor started to prescribe and stopped since it is now available over the counter; the fact is that insurance companies are unlikely to pay for a drug that's available over the counter. "The insurance companies might abandon their patients who need this drug. That could be very problematic to many patients who can't afford it," says Dr. Peter J. Baiocco, associate chief of the gastroenterology section at Lenox Hill Hospital in New York City. Doctors already have to provide extra information to insurance companies when they want to prescribe Prilosec to a patient for more than a couple of months, said Baiocco.

Gastroenterologists say some patients do have to take Prilosec each day—typically one pill—to treat chronic heartburn. If insurance companies don't pay, that could add up to more than $300 a year, much more than proven herbal remedies. After all, there's a lot of advertising to pay for.

If It's on TV, It Must Be True

Lets' face it. We are a culture depending on—and convinced of—the "healthy" practice of taking drugs. As our friend found out while waiting for his prescriptions, television commercial breaks are in no shortage of ads pushing pharmaceutical drugs. And these ads all have the same basic message: "Feel bad? Take our drug and feel good." Is that why the media always touts new unproven drugs, and rarely mentions prescription drug deaths or alternative therapies for health?

In 2000, pharmaceutical companies spent $2.5 billion on mass media ads for prescription drugs. Admittedly, this is a small portion of the $101.6 billion spent on advertising of mainstream consumer products in the United States. But consider the following:

- PepsiCo spent $125 million advertising Pepsi Cola—less than the $160 million Merck spent advertising Vioxx to consumers.
- Vioxx also beat out Budweiser's beer ad campaign of $146 million and was close to the most heavily advertised car—GM's Saturn—with ad spending of $169 million in 2000.
- Each of the top seven most heavily advertised prescription drugs beat Nike's ad budget of $78.2 million for its shoes.
- More was spent on advertising in each of the top fifteen individual drugs than Campbell's $58 million for its soups.

The bottom line? Drugs are as much a pedestrian part of our existence as is our lunchtime soup or the shoes we wear.

Increasing Spending on Prescription Drugs

Spending on prescription drugs escalated more than 12 percent per year in five of the eight years between 1993 and 2000. Spending on retail prescription drugs increased 18.8 percent from 1999 to 2000 and is anticipated that the increase will continue to be between 15 and 20 percent annually for the foreseeable future.

The dramatic rise in spending on prescription drugs can be attributed to a few related factors. In 1992 there were roughly 1.9 billion prescriptions dispensed in the United States, and in 2000 there were 2.9 billion. Americans are demanding, and physicians are prescribing, a higher volume of medicines each year. The rising volume of prescriptions is driven by three factors:

- an increase in the general U.S. population and the aging of the population
- an increase in number of people being prescribed drug therapy
- an increase in the number of prescriptions per person

The average number of prescriptions per person in the United States increased from 7.3 in 1992 to 10.4 in 2000. Along with this increase in demand, there has been a shift toward the use of more expensive medications. It's more than a coincidence that many of the most expensive medications happen to be those medications that are most heavily advertised.

About half of the increase in retail drug spending between 1999 and 2000 occurred among just eight drug classes—anti-hypertensives, antilipemics, COX-II inhibitors, antidepressants, proton pump inhibitors, antidiabetics, antiepileptics, and pain relievers. Major drugs in these classes are extensively advertised both to prescribing physicians and directly to consumers. Interestingly, the ten drugs with the heaviest direct-to-consumer advertising accounted for 34 percent of the total increase in spending. Those drugs will probably sound familiar. They include:

- Vioxx and Celebrex (COX-II inhibitors)
- Claritin and Allegra (for allergies)
- Paxil (for depression)
- Prilosec and Prevacid (for GERD)
- Zocor and Pravachol (for hyperlipidemia)
- Viagra (for erectile dysfunction)

Based upon the dramatic increases in spending for heavily advertised drugs, it is evident that the consumer advertising campaigns are working very well.

How many ads for dietary supplements like multivitamins have you ever seen on TV—or ephedra for that matter? (Infomercials for coral calcium on cable TV don't count!) More than likely it's been few, if any.

If you remember our patient selected a weight loss product containing the ephedra substitute synephrine. The fact is, there's much less evidence about synephrine's health benefits and safety than there is about ephedra, which *has* been heavily studied. In fact, no one really knows if there are risks with ingesting synephrine or not. But hey, the important thing is that it's not that dangerous herb ephedra, right?

Food Fights

As I mentioned earlier, the FDA also has control over approving new foods and ingredients. Do you remember how the patient in our scenario passed by the low-fat potato chips in the food section of the pharmacy? Let's examine the case of the fat substitute olestra. When first announced, many people were excited about olestra because of the possibility it could assist people in eating diets lower in saturated and overall fat—and thereby prevent obesity and heart disease.

But there were some problems. Simply put, olestra causes gastrointestinal disturbances (which are sometimes severe), including diarrhea, fecal urgency, and more frequent and looser bowel movements. (Some reports also described olestra's cause of "underwear staining" associated with "anal leakage.") The Center for Science in the Public Interest (CSPI) reports that a variety of gastrointestinal symptoms occurred in subjects who consumed on a daily basis the amount of olestra that would be found in less than one ounce of potato chips (about 16 chips), as well as higher doses.

Data is lacking on the health effects of olestra on potentially vulnerable segments of the population. Key tests were unacceptably brief. According to the CSPI, "Only poor studies have examined the effect of olestra on gastrointestinal disturbances in children, while no studies at all have focused on gastrointestinal problems and nutrient loss in healthy people over forty-four years of age and people with poor nutritional status."

Doesn't sound to me like something you'd want to serve at your next Super Bowl party.

Sweet Stuff

You might recall that our imaginary patient bought the sugar substitute aspartame—commonly known by the brand names NutraSweet and Equal—to reduce his intake of sugar calories. Good thought, but probably the wrong solution. In 1996, Ralph G. Walton, M.D., Chairman of the Center for Behavioral Medicine, Northeastern Ohio Universities College of Medicine, conducted a survey of peer-reviewed medical literature about the safety of aspartame using various research databases. Dr. Walton analyzed 164 studies which he believed were related to human safety questions. Of those studies, seventy-four studies had aspartame industry-related sponsorship and ninety were funded without any industry money.

Of the seventy-four aspartame industry-sponsored studies, all seventy-four (100 percent) claimed that no problems were found with aspartame. Of the ninety non-industry-sponsored studies, eighty-three (92 percent) identified one or more problems with aspartame. Of the seven studies which did not find a problem, six of those studies were conducted by the FDA. Given that a number of FDA officials went to work for the aspartame industry immediately following approval (including the former FDA Commissioner), many consider these studies to be equivalent to industry-sponsored research.

Now let's contrast the story of aspartame with that of another sweetener, commonly called stevia. If you go to your local health food store, you will probably find a stevia product (scientific name *Stevia rebaudiana*) on the shelves. Originating in various parts of Asia and South America, stevia is commonly used throughout the rest of the world. Why? Well, it's easy to grow, it's cheap, and most of all, it's up to three hundred times sweeter than table sugar. And best of all, it has no calories.

Unlike most of us, the FDA most definitely has heard of stevia. In 1991 the FDA blocked the importation of stevia leaves and extracts. In 1995, they issued a revision which allowed stevia leaves or stevioside extracts to be imported if explicitly labeled as a dietary supplement or for use as an ingredient of a dietary supplement. However, it is not allowed to be imported or used as a commercial sweetener or flavoring agent. You usually have to go to a health food store to find it. Though commonplace in countries throughout the world, here it is labeled as a "supplement," and can't be called an "additive" or "food." Since the mid-1980s, the FDA has labeled stevia an "unsafe food additive" and gone to extensive lengths to keep it off the U.S. market—including initiating a search-and-seizure campaign and full-fledged "import alert."

Is stevia dangerous? To judge from the extensive measures the FDA has employed to keep stevia away from the public, one might think so. The truth is, no ill effects have ever been found. However, the FDA has remained so adamant on the subject that even though stevia can now be legally marketed as a dietary supplement under legislation enacted in 1994, any mention of its possible use as a sweetener or tea is still strictly prohibited. To top things off, since stevia has been designated as "unsafe"—almost certainly to benefit the politically powerful sweetener industry—the agency has insisted on stonewalling any and all evidence to the contrary.

As Rob McCaleb, president and founder of the Herb Research Foundation, has said, "Sweetness is big money." In other words, the powers that be don't want to see a product that is cheap and easy to grow on the market competing with their own products.

Finally, there's one other point in our scenario that requires mentioning; the vitamin with "500 percent more of the nutrient than recommended." We can't blame the FDA for this one. Instead this is the handiwork of the U.S. Department of Agriculture (USDA), although some would argue this area—the determination of nutritional standards—should fall under the FDA. Simply put, the 500 percent figure is the amount above the minimum daily requirement and has nothing to due with toxicity. Many experts argue that these "minimum daily requirements" (what were once called RDAs and now called DRIs) are woefully inadequate. Therefore, we have need of higher intake of various nutrients. Either way, it's very unlikely that you'll suffer drastic side effects from taking a multivitamin. (For more information on this topic, see Woodland Publishing's *Real RDAs for Real People*.)

Well, I suspect I've spooked you at least a little about the regulatory problems at the FDA. If so, good! It is important for us to understand both the regulatory and political climate that exists within the FDA as it decides whether to ban or severely limit the sale of ephedra products.

At this point you might be asking yourself any number of questions: "Is the FDA doing the right thing in asking for more information?" "Is the negative chorus against ephedra realistic, or is it motivated by more than the public's safety?" "Why is the FDA dragging its feet in taking definitive action for or against ephedra?" "What role does the dietary supplement industry play in all this?" And finally, "Is this entire uproar only about ephedra, or is there a bigger picture here?"

You'll find the answers to these questions and more in the following chapters.

CHAPTER 4

In Defense of Ephedra

"AT THE TIME MR. BECHLER collapsed from heat stroke, much of the ephedrine he had swallowed was still in his stomach and had not yet entered his bloodstream. [The unabsorbed ephedrine] could not have caused or contributed to Mr. Bechler's death."

> – *Forensic pathologist Dr. Michael Baden, former New York City chief medical examiner, in a letter to the Subcommittee on Oversight and Investigations Hearing on Issues Relating to Ephedra-Containing Dietary Supplements, July 23, 2003*

In August 2000, a group of scientists, government officials, industry experts and interested parties gathered at the Office of Women's Health (OWH), a part of the Department of Health and Human Services (HHS). They were in Washington, D.C. for two days of hearings about the safety and risks of ephedrine alkaloids. The FDA and the Center for Food Safety and Applied Nutrition (CFSAN) sponsored the meeting.

The hearings were spurred by the FDA's recent change in its proposed policy announced in 1997, which would have drastically curtailed the use of ephedra. Specifically, the proposal called for limiting intake of ephedra to 8 mg of total ephedra alkaloids per dosage, and a total daily dosage of 24 mg for a duration of use not to exceed seven days. It also required an extensive warning label, banned any combinations with products containing caffeine or other stimulants, and prohibited any claims that would encourage use for more than seven days, including claims for weight loss or sports performance. The FDA claimed that its proposed rules were based in part on hundreds of adverse event reports (AERs) associated with the use of ephedra—including alleged deaths—received by the agency.

After a flurry of complaints from Congress and the dietary supplement industry over the scientific accuracy of the safety data supporting FDA's position of stricter controls, the FDA withdrew its proposal. The clincher was a report from the General Accounting Office (GAO) criticizing the manner in which the FDA's policy was developed, especially the adverse event reports allegedly associated with ephedra.

When the GAO report came out, members of Congress were appalled. "I am concerned about the apparent lack of scientific data behind the FDA's actions," said House Science Committee Chairman F. James Sensenbrenner, Jr. (R-WI). "For the FDA—one of the most important regulatory agencies in government—to use such poor science for a dietary supplement raises warning flags for the other products the agency regulates."

There were similar comments from the other side of the aisle. "According to the GAO report, FDA missed the mark in their proposed regulation," said Congressman Ralph Hall (D-TX). "Documentation of FDA's work was inadequate, they failed to record key steps in their analysis, they neglected to review the AERs for reliability, they arbitrarily inflated the benefits of their regulation and all of this fed into their proposed rule." Hall added, "I would suggest that FDA withdraw the proposed rule, do their job right and see whether we can't come up with a rule that everyone can support grounded in real science and reliable data."

The GAO found that the FDA's rule-making regarding ephedrine alkaloids relied almost exclusively on adverse event reports (AERs) that were not reviewed for linkage to ephedra or for reliability by the FDA. For example, the FDA relied on just thirteen AERs as the "sole source of support for specific dosing levels," yet the GAO described those critical AERs as "poorly documented." Examining the thirteen AERs, the GAO noted that, among other problems, three AERs included reports where the physician explicitly noted that the cause of the event was not related to dietary supplements. The GAO added that the FDA, "did not perform a causal analysis to determine if, in fact, the thirteen AERs it used to set dosing levels were caused by supplements containing ephedrine alkaloids."

On February 25, 2000, the FDA associate commissioner for legislation, Melinda K. Plaisier, sent a letter to members of Congress concerned with drug and dietary supplement regulation announcing the agency planned another attempt to evaluate the "the potential health risks associated with those products." CFSAN's Joseph Levitt described the withdrawal as a "mid-course correction" and not a surrender or capitulation. Levitt noted that the agency had new information to review, that it would hold a public hearing, and "follow that data, wherever it leads us."

Then, on April 3, 2000, the FDA released a report entitled "Assessment of Public Health Risks Associated with the Use of Ephedrine Alkaloid-Containing Dietary Supplements." In the report, the FDA used four types of evidence to show that the unrestricted use of ephedrine constituted an ongoing public health menace:

• A summary of 140 adverse event reports (AERs) submitted between June 1, 1997 and March 1, 1999, which purport to demonstrate medical complications caused by ephedrine

- A systematic analysis of these AERs
- A literature review summarizing the existing peer-reviewed literature on ephedra toxicity
- An analysis of the first three items provided by a panel of independent reviewers

After reviewing the accumulated data, FDA analysts felt there was a clear connection to ephedrine alkaloids in sixty of the cases, approximately one-third of which involved the cardiovascular system. The sixty cases were submitted to medical reviewers who analyzed them separately, and then jointly, before determining that a connection existed between the episode described and the use of ephedrine alkaloids.

What the FDA *did not* refer to was criticism leveled at it a year earlier during a hearing of the Committee on Government Reform. Congressman Dan Burton (R-IN) indicated his committee identified six problem areas in the FDA's adverse events monitoring systems, including "causality not established." Burton said, "Ironically, this is done for veterinary drugs. For instance, if a dog takes a medicine and a dog has a heart attack and dies, the FDA evaluates this report to see if the death was related to the drug or not. . . . With people and dietary supplement events, the FDA has not done this analysis."

Representative Burton brought up two specific cases regarding ephedra. He pointed out that one death attributed to ephedra was actually attributable to hypothermia. The other was the death of a woman who had been using an ephedra supplement and who died after driving her automobile the wrong way on a one-way street and striking a pole going 90 miles an hour. "Her blood alcohol limit was .212, more than twice the legally intoxicated limit in most states," said Burton. "Are these two cases really ephedra deaths?"

Now, back to the hearings at the Office of Women's Health. Some people suspected the FDA might have orchestrated the meetings to give it an excuse to remove ephedra from the market. Their fears lay specifically in the fact that under the Dietary Supplement Health and Education Act of 1994 (DSHEA), the FDA has the authority to pull an unsafe dietary supplement from the market if the Secretary of Health and Human Services—and not the FDA Commissioner (who reports to the Secretary of HHS)—deems it an "imminent hazard" to public health, as long as HHS can justify its actions in an administrative hearing. If the recommendations by OWH, based on testimony provided at the hearing, convinced the Secretary that ephedra dietary supplements posed an imminent hazard, then at least some of the procedural requirements for removal might be met and therefore doom ephedra.

Whether that was a formal strategy or just paranoia, we'll never know. If it was a strategy, testimony presented at the hearing provided a more difficult challenge than the folks involved had anticipated.

A panel at the meeting, comprised of a group of seven scientists hired by the Ephedra Education Council (EEC), reported its findings after performing a comprehensive review of all the studies to date, along with the AERs compiled by the FDA.

And what did the seven scientists report? They clearly stated that there was no supporting data proving a link between the use of dietary supplements containing ephedrine alkaloids and serious adverse events when used according to the recommendations made by the industry. These recommendations included:

- Serving limits of no more than 25 mg of total ephedrine alkaloids
- Limits on daily consumption of not more than 100 mg of total ephedrine alkaloids
- Appropriate warnings consistent with other available over-the-counter ephedrine alkaloid products (See the sidebar "What is Meant by 'Adverse Event'?" for complete statement.)

Maybe you're thinking, "Ah-hah! What would you expect people hired by the ephedra lobby group to say?" However, it's important to point out a few things. First, they have been completely above board about their relationship—nothing, as far as I have been able to determine, has been hidden or subverted; no scientists have been pulled off the panel because they disagree with the industry (at least as far as I discovered); and they've laid out their credentials—and reputations—for all to see. The panel included the following experts:

- *Stephen E. Kimmel, M.D.* An expert in cardiovascular epidemiology from the University of Pennsylvania, Dr. Kimmel is a leading researcher in the effect of drugs on the heart.
- *Stephen B. Karch, M.D.* Dr. Karch is a cardiac pathologist and medical examiner from San Francisco with specific expertise in the cardiac toxicity of catecholamines, including ephedrine and ephedrine alkaloids derived from ephedra.
- *Norbert P. Page, M.S., D.V.M.* Dr. Page has thirty years experience in chemical and radiation toxicology, and was previously Director of Scientific Affairs for Toxic Substances and Pesticides at the EPA and Director of the NCI's Carcinogen Testing Program.
- *Theodore Farber, Ph.D., D.A.B.T.* Dr. Farber has over twenty years of experience as a toxicologist and pharmacologist with the federal government, including senior positions as the Director of the Division of Drug and Environmental Toxicology in the Center for Veterinary Medicine at FDA and the Director of the Health Effects Division at EPA.
- *John W. Olney, M.D.* A leading researcher in the effects of food ingredients and other chemicals on the brain from Washington University Medical School in St. Louis.
- *Grover M. Hutchins, M.D.* A researcher and author in pathology and cardiac pathology from John Hopkins University.
- *Edgar H. Adams, M.S., Sc.D.* An expert in substance abuse, Dr. Adams worked for seventeen years at the National Institute on Drug Abuse (NIDA), during which time he supervised several data collection and analysis initiatives as the

head of the Division of Epidemiology and Prevention Research, including the Drug Abuse Warning Network (DAWN) and the National Household Survey on Drug Abuse.

After studying the AERs the FDA submitted in April, one of the EEC Expert Panel members, Steven B. Karch, M.D., noted that a detailed review of all four elements clearly showed the FDA had failed to make a case for the toxicity of ephedra-containing dietary supplements—though it has made a stronger case against over-the-counter (OTC) drugs such as phenyl-propanolamine (PPA) and pseudoephedrine (PE). PPA is an ingredient used in prescription and OTC nasal decongestant and appetite-control drug products. PE is a common decongestant in a variety of cold and cough products.

Along with Drs. Page and Farber, Dr. Karch prepared an analysis of the entire case series where he dealt only with FDA claims of cardiovascular toxicity. Dr. Karch said two general considerations about AERs were important enough to mention. The first is the AER system itself. The detection of adverse drug reactions has traditionally been the role of the medical community and of peer-reviewed medical journals. He said from his experience, the medical community is usually more observant than any government agency, and very few case reports describing ephedrine-related toxicity have been published in the peer-reviewed medical literature.

He said one explanation for the disparity in the number of case reports published in peer-reviewed journals and the very large number of case reports received by the FDA is papers submitted to peer-reviewed medical journals are scrutinized far more critically than those submitted to the FDA.

Dr. Karch said an equally plausible explanation is significant numbers of ephedrine-related complications are simply not occurring, and therefore no one is writing papers about them. The likelihood of the alternate explanation is reinforced by the lack of evidence to be found in government surveys not commissioned by the FDA, particularly surveillance of drug abuse patterns and complications sponsored by the Substance Abuse and Mental Health Services Administration (SAMHSA). "Neither the Medical Examiner nor the Emergency Room (ER) components of the Drug Abuse Warning Network (DAWN), nor the National Household Drug Abuse Survey (NHDAS) contain any data suggesting that ephedrine toxicity is nearly the problem which FDA perceives it to be," said Dr. Karch.

Dr. Karch noted that of the fourteen reported cases of cardiac arrest, the FDA panel placed only four in the "attributable" or "supporting" groups. In three of these four cases, other much more plausible explanations for the adverse event seemed the likely cause. In one case, that of a dieting and overweight woman who had been fasting, vital information (her electrolyte status) was never reported. Case by case, the panel showed how the FDA confusion, inaccuracy and outright errors undermined the whole AER set. As for the literature cited, Dr. Karch said it "consists of many references that are either irrelevant or inappropriate to an analysis of the safety of ephedra products."

One citation was not even a case report. Instead, it was a letter to the editor describing a case where an episode of angina was thought to have been the result of pseudoephedrine (PE) ingestion. Of the eight cases the FDA presented to prove that ephedrine caused angina and/or infarction, there was only one ephedrine case cited—that of a chronic ephedrine abuser.

Dr. Stephen E. Kimmel, the panel's chair, summarized his group's findings: "Conservative estimates suggest no greater risk for adverse events than the risk in the general population," he continued. "The number of reported adverse events are consistent with what would occur in the general population, even after accounting for possible under-reporting of events. Such findings represent the efforts of the panel to step back from the emotional impact that individual adverse reports can have and look objectively at the available scientific information."

Not really what the FDA wanted to hear, wouldn't you say?

The EEC panel members weren't the only ones who found ephedra to be safe. George Bray, Boyd Professor of Medicine at Louisiana State University and Executive Director of the Pennington Biomedical Research Center, discussed the results of completed clinical trials that show that dietary supplements containing ephedrine alkaloids are effective and safe as weight loss products. "I am here today to argue for the continued availability of over-the-counter products containing ephedra alkaloids as one tool to help combat obesity," said Dr. Bray.

He reported that, in his view, ephedra products offered a safe, effective and affordable option for losing weight. He concluded that, "the balance of the risk-benefit fulcrum is clearly on the side of benefit."

Nothing Rotten About Ephedra in Denmark

Dr. Arne Astrup of Copenhagen, Denmark, a well-respected researcher in the treatment of obesity, discussed data from his own research supporting the safety and efficacy of ephedrine/caffeine combinations in weight loss. Dr. Astrup's studies of ephedrine and caffeine found that the combination proved effective as a weight-loss product.

Dr. Astrup also pointed to an FDA report on the published literature as misrepresenting data in his study on the safety of the two ingredients to instead support FDA's allegations concerning ephedra. "I think our data and results are mischaracterized and the presentation is flawed and distorted," said Dr. Astrup. "It's giving a very negative picture of the safety profile of the combination of ephedrine/caffeine, which is not supported by our research."

More experts provided evidence in support of ephedra. Drs. Patricia A. Daly and Carol Boozer, who conducted two clinical trials of ephedra/caffeine combination products at hospitals associated with Harvard and Columbia Universities, presented data from an eight-week study showing that ephedra products could produce safe and significant weight loss. They also announced that a longer-term, more comprehensive follow-up study had been completed and was currently being prepared for publication. These researchers reported that there were no serious adverse events seen in their latest study.

There were also consumers and several treating physicians who testified as to their experience and success using ephedra products for weight loss. One was Ms. Mario Banks, a school teacher from Jasper, Alabama. "I am proof that ephedra-based products are indeed a safe, simple and reliable program for losing and maintaining weight loss," said Ms. Banks. "In four months I am thrilled to be thirty pounds lighter. This has just been a wonderful and positive experience."

Dr. Gary Huber of the Texas Nutrition Institute reported on his own research data on ephedra used alone or in combination with caffeine that these products are safe and effective for weight loss. Dr. Huber was accompanied by three patients who recounted their personal experiences with the products and the physical and mental health benefits that resulted from their loss of weight.

Varying Amounts

Ephedra doses in the studies presented during the hearings varied between 8 to 25 mg total alkaloids per dose, ranging between 72 to 150 mg total per day; sometimes in combination with caffeine, sometimes not. There was a consensus that larger, randomized controlled clinical trials for weight loss, endurance and body building were needed. They noted the few trials and studies reported at the meeting consisted primarily of small groups—fewer than 150 people, and of short durations of use—between six and eight weeks. They also noted that data on long-term weight loss and maintenance were scarce and might have as much to do with calorie-restricted diets as the ephedra products themselves.

A Call to Action? No, Inaction

Based on the statement issued by Dr. Wanda Jones, Deputy Assistant Secretary for Women's Health at NIH, things didn't seem quite as dire as we hear today. "The available evidence for adverse effects, particularly from the adverse event reports (AERs) submitted to FDA, is very circumstantial," said Dr. Jones. "While these reported adverse events give cause for concern, the AER data set is not robust."

Jones noted that experts at the meeting pointed out inherent weaknesses of a passive reporting system. Also, while some rare adverse events "plausibly and temporally" might be related to use of ephedrine alkaloids, she noted that opinion was divided on the value of the AER system in assessing the strength of the association. "Information presented at, and contained in the transcript of, this meeting indicates a need for enhanced AER capability, including engaging industry to improve the quality of the system."

In her concluding remarks, Dr. Jones added, "Given the current widespread use of EADS [ephedrine alkaloid dietary supplements], a consumer education campaign about these products is warranted. Good manufacturing standards are needed, reasonable dose and duration levels determined, and warnings and contraindications clearly indicated on labels." She added, "A research agenda should be established. Therefore, the research community should take the next logical step by conducting a systematic review of the world's literature on ephedra."

Jones recommended that after compiling the state of the science and identifying the limitations and gaps of the current research, an appropriate agenda could be established. "In this regard, the National Center for Complementary and Alternative Medicine of the National Institutes of Health already is requesting proposals to study herb-drug interactions," said Jones.

A few presenters suggested the results of newer studies to be published the following year might show EADS to be effective and safe—or not—for short-term weight loss, but there were no large-scale studies forthcoming.

Soon after the meeting, an industry coalition of four leading dietary supplement trade associations formally petitioned the FDA to adopt a national standard for the labeling of dietary supplements containing ephedra. The petition was filed on October 25, 2000 by the American Herbal Products Association (AHPA), Consumer Healthcare Products Association (CHPA), National Nutritional Foods Association (NNFA) and the Utah Natural Products Alliance (UNPA)—organizations whose members comprise many of the manufacturers and distributors of dietary supplements containing ephedra.

The group also suggested that the current industry label warning of ephedra be adopted as the official national standard. The label states the following:

> Warning: Not intended for use by anyone under the age of 18. Do not use this product if you are pregnant or nursing. Consult a health care professional before using this product if you have heart disease, thyroid disease, diabetes, high blood pressure, depression or other psychiatric condition, glaucoma, difficulty in urinating, prostate enlargement, or seizure disorder, if you are using a monoamine oxidase inhibitor (MAOI), or any other prescription drug, or you are using an over-the-counter drug containing ephedrine, pseudoephedrine or phenylpropanolamine (ingredients found in certain allergy, asthma, cough/cold and weight-control products).
>
> Exceeding recommended serving will not improve results and may cause serious adverse health effects.

Discontinue use and call a health care professional immediately if you experience rapid heartbeat, dizziness, severe headache, shortness of breath, or other similar symptoms."

Journal Entries

Seven months after the hearings at the Office of Women's Health, the Boozer-Daly clinical study appeared in the March 2001 issue of the peer-reviewed *International Journal of Obesity*. The study showed a commercial product, Metabolife 356, produced significant weight loss over an eight-week period. The study, conducted by researchers from St. Luke's Roosevelt Hospital Center and the department of Medicine at Columbia School of Medicine, included sixty-seven subjects with thirty-two taking a placebo and the rest taking 73 mg a day of ephedrine alkaloids and 240 mg per day of caffeine from guarana.

The researchers concluded the ephedrine-caffeine combination did, indeed, promote short-term weight loss—an average of 4 kg for the treatment group—but recommended further studies be conducted to determine if there would be sustained weight loss over a longer term.

During the study, none of the placebo group withdrew, while eight of the treatment group did. The most common reasons for withdrawal were dry mouth, headache and insomnia. Funding was provided by Science Toxicology and Technology Consulting, Metabolife, and a National Institute of Health (NIH) grant.

This is probably a good place to discuss AERs a little more. Shortly after the Boozer-Daly study came out, the FDA released a statement on the AER issue regarding ephedra. The seven-member panel agreed with their findings: in essence, that there was no proven association between ephedra consumption and serious adverse events (AERs).

Basically, they said AERs cannot be viewed as scientific "data," and it is not possible to use AERs to establish whether an event is attributable to ephedra, or whether ephedra increases the risk of adverse events. They also said the industry would be willing to review all new AERs that the FDA receives for ephedra products in an effort to help monitor whether the current national standard for these products is working, which they hoped would promote a more cooperative approach with the FDA concerning the regulation of the supplements.

"These conclusions are also consistent with a quantitative risk study submitted to the FDA in December 2000 by Cantox Health Sciences International, and with data from clinical studies on ephedrine and ephedra products, including the recently published abstract of the Harvard and Columbia study," added Dr. Kimmel, one of the "EEC 7."

Oh, Canada!

The "Cantox Report," was the first formal risk assessment on dietary supplements containing ephedra and ephedra alkaloids. Who is Cantox? Canadian-based Cantox Health Sciences International provides scientific consulting services, specializing in safety and regulatory issues related to products and processes affecting human health and the environment. For more than twenty years, Cantox has worked with clients and projects in over 100 countries. Cantox's President, Ian Munro, Ph.D., is a regulatory toxicologist and Chairman of the UL Subcommittee, Food and Nutrition Board (FNB), U.S. National Academies. Cantox's principal investigator on the ephedra risk assessment project was Earle Nestmann, Ph.D., a recognized authority in toxicology with extensive experience in regulatory issues and risk assessment. The ephedra risk assessment was contracted and funded by the Council for Responsible Nutrition (CRN), which in turn is funded by a broad spectrum of companies, not only firms selling ephedra products.

The objective of the Cantox Report was to perform a quantitative risk assessment for the botanical ephedra as used in dietary supplements, which involved a review and interpretation of all data sources and determination of an Upper Limit (UL) for ephedrine alkaloids in ephedra. This was done through application of the Tolerable Upper Intake Level (also called Upper Limit, or UL) method developed by the Food and Nutrition Board, Institute of Medicine, National Academies for application to nutrients. It was not the purpose of the study to perform a risk-benefit analysis.

Based on the evidence, particularly the results of nineteen relevant clinical trials, including the preliminary results of the Boozer study scheduled to appear in the March 2001 issue of the *International Journal of Obesity*, the Cantox study pegged the "No Observed Adverse Effect Level" (NOAEL) for ephedra at 90 mg per day taken in three equal doses of 30 mg. And the "Lowest Observed Adverse Effect Level" (LOAEL) was set at 150 mg per day. At these levels, they found the adverse effects were of "moderate intensity and are not life-threatening or debilitating."

They found that the AERs were not conclusive, they were not useful in identifying limits because they did not prove blame, and therefore were not an adequate basis for identifying appropriate limits. They found the overall rate of adverse effects was low, considering the amount of ephedra sold and consumed.

The Cantox Report determined there were other factors in the AERs that made them less reliable:

• Most of the reports focused on the product identity and characterization of the adverse event.
• Many contained little information of reliable quality.
• Others lacked critical information needed for any possible assignment of cause.

- Most reports lacked reliable dosage information.
- Some are confounded by preexisting conditions and others by concomitant intakes of other substances that may have caused or contributed to the adverse effect.

Based on the scientific evidence, Cantox also made recommendations for the safe use of ephedra supplements, including:

- Dosage limits of 90 mg per day, with no more than 30 mg per dose
- Labeling to provide exclusions and contraindications consistent with the nineteen clinical trials that are the basis of the upper limit (UL)
- Label statement that encourages user to check with health care provider about use
- Limit use to six months or less
- Not for anyone younger than eighteen years old
- Postmarket monitoring

In defense of the FDA, in April 2001 the Office of Inspector General, which is part of HHS, reported that unlike new prescription and over-the-counter drugs, the FDA does not have the authority to require supplements to undergo premarket approval for safety and efficacy. Instead, it relies mostly on its adverse event reporting system to identify safety problems.

The Office of Inspector General said the FDA's Adverse Event Reporting System for Dietary Supplements is flawed partially because reporting adverse events is entirely voluntary. The report admitted the FDA's adverse event reporting system detects only a small portion of the events that actually occur. It stated a recent FDA-commissioned study estimated that the FDA receives less than 1 percent of all adverse events associated with dietary supplements. Among the factors that may contribute to under-reporting are that many consumers presume supplements to be safe, use these products without the supervision of a health care professional, and may be unaware that the FDA regulates them. The FDA's limited outreach concerning this system contributes to this unawareness. It has difficulty generating signals of possible public health concerns. The FDA lacks much of the information that is necessary to effectively analyze adverse event reports and to generate possible signals of concern.

We Report, You Concur

After the FDA and Cantox reports came out, the seven-member EEC panel pointed out why, as with past reports, this batch of AERs shows why frequent media reporting of the raw number of AERs is meaningless and only confuses consumers. (Just think of the headlines after baseball player Steve Bechler died, on which we'll have more in the next chapter.)

The researchers found the AERs included had no relationship to ephedra use. Included were reports on products that did not contain ephedra, reports where no adverse event was even listed, and cases where the event occurred well prior to any ephedra consumption. Also included were cases medically unrelated to ephedra, such as gallstones, small bowel obstruction and fat feet, as well as absurd reports including one where a married woman had an affair with a student, and blamed ephedra for her behavior. She eventually was criminally prosecuted.

The only experts who have reviewed the entire FDA collection of AERs have consistently found that the AERs, when considered in the context of scientific data from clinical studies, do not represent a public health concern when ephedra products did not exceed 90–100 mg per day.

The EEC panel went even further. They claimed that not only did independent researchers and leading academic experts consulting with industry prove the AER database was not useful

from a scientific standpoint, but also that the FDA had seriously mischaracterized the published literature. They also claimed
that the FDA and its consultants had ignored data regarding the
benefits of these products.

Back to the Lab

A year later, some of the same researchers involved in the
March 2001 clinical study reported above published new find-
ings after a six-month trial of ephedra use. Appearing in the
April 2002 issue of the *International Journal of Obesity,* the
researchers described it as "the first reported long-term, clinical
trial of a herbal preparation containing ephedrine alkaloids and
caffeine in combination." The researchers involved including
Dr. Carol Boozer, the director of the New York Obesity
Research Center at St. Luke's-Roosevelt Hospital and Columbia
University, and Dr. Patricia Daly, formerly a professor at Beth
Israel Medical Center at Harvard Medical School.

The study followed thorough protocols; it was a prospective,
two-arm, six-month, randomized, double-blind, placebo-controlled, clinical safety and efficacy trial conducted at two sites.

Recruited for the study were 167 overweight subjects, with
eighty-four assigned to the placebo group and the remaining
eighty-three assigned to the ephedra/caffeine alkaloid group.
For six months, the subjects were given daily either a placebo
or 90 mg of ephedrine alkaloids (from herbal ephedra) and 192
mg of caffeine alkaloids (from kola nut) in three divided doses,
along with diet and exercise counseling. All the subjects were
instructed to eat normally—but to limit intake of dietary fat to
30 percent of calories—and to exercise thirty minutes per day,
three times a week for exercise.

The subjects underwent twenty-four-hour blood pressure and
cardiac Holter monitoring (which shows the electrical activity
of your heart, including rate, rhythm and whether your heart is

beating correctly), as well as EKGs, routine laboratory tests, and urine samples. The researchers said that during the study, there were a similar number of subjects in both groups who dropped out because of potential adverse effects. Of the eighty subjects who withdrew from the study, thirty-seven were from the treated group and forty-three were from the placebo group. Less than half of the withdrawals in both groups were related to side effects.

After the study was completed, the researchers found that compared with placebo, the tested product produced no adverse events and minimal side effects consistent with the known action mechanisms of ephedrine and caffeine. They also noted there were "no significant differences between treatment groups in self-reported chest pain, palpitations, blurred vision, headache, nausea or irritability at any point."

None of the subjects suffered from a serious adverse event, and the side effects in both groups were transient and mild. The researchers noted that "the symptoms that subjects reported to be most consistently increased by the herbal vs. the placebo treatment were dry mouth, heartburn and insomnia."

And what about the weight loss? The researchers concluded that "herbal ephedra/caffeine (90/192 mg/day) promoted body weight and body fat rejection and improved blood lipids without significant adverse events."

The researchers also concluded that "herbal ephedra/caffeine herbal supplements, when used as directed by healthy overweight men and women in combination with healthy diet and exercise habits, may be beneficial for weight reduction without significantly increased risk of adverse events. The current widespread usage of herbal products and the increasing incidence of obesity warrant additional clinical trials to confirm and extend these results."

I thought a note on Dr. Boozer's background might be helpful, since she will be mentioned again in the next chapter. Dr. Boozer is a nutrition scientist with primary research interests in the area of energy metabolism. She received her doctorate from Harvard (School of Public Health). In 1994, she joined the New York Obesity Research Center with an appointment to Assistant Professor of Nutrition at the Institute of Human Nutrition, Columbia University. Her research is supported primarily by grants from the National Institutes of Health (NIH), with some secondary funding from industry. She is active in several professional organizations and is currently the Membership Chair of the North American Association for the Study of Obesity.

The Bomb Shell

On February 28, 2003, the Department of Health and Human Services (HHS) issued a press release titled, "HHS Acts to Reduce Safety Concerns Associated with Dietary Supplements Containing Ephedra." In the statement, the HHS said based on new evidence, including a study by the RAND Corporation, that dietary supplements containing ephedra *"may present significant or unreasonable risks as currently marketed,"* and announced a series of actions designed to protect Americans from these risks (emphasis added).

To this end, the FDA said it sought public comment on:

• The new evidence on health risks associated with ephedra, to establish an up-to-date public record as quickly as possible to support any appropriate new restrictions on ephedra-containing products.
• Whether the currently available evidence and medical literature present a "significant or unreasonable risk of illness or injury" from dietary supplements containing ephedra. This is the standard that must be met under the Dietary Supplement Health and Education Act for the government to take regulatory action on ephedra.

- A strong new warning label on any ephedra products that continue to be marketed. The proposed label warns about reports of serious adverse events after use of ephedra, including heart attack, seizure, stroke, and death; cautions that the risk can increase with the dose, with strenuous exercise, and with other stimulants such as caffeine; specifies certain groups (such as women who are pregnant or breast feeding and persons under eighteen) who should not use these products; and lists other diseases, such as heart disease and high blood pressure, that should rule out the use of ephedrine alkaloids.
- Issuing a set of warning letters against ephedra products making unsubstantiated claims about sports performance enhancement. The RAND study found only minimal scientific evidence in support of such health claims.

Huh? I have read the RAND report and that's not what it says. Perhaps a little background would be helpful.

The RAND report, commissioned by the National Institutes of Health, reviewed recent evidence on the risks and benefits of ephedra and ephedrine. After searching published reports, journal articles, conference presentations, and various sources of unpublished studies, they identified fifty-two controlled clinical trials of ephedrine or herbal ephedra for weight loss or athletic performance in humans. The FDA provided them with copies of over one thousand adverse event reports (AERs) related to herbal ephedra and 125 AERs related to ephedrine. These reports often included interviews with patients and/or family members, extensive medical records, and copies of product labels. They also identified sixty-five case reports in the literature and received a disk of 15,951 reports containing 18,502 cases from Metabolife, a prominent manufacturer of ephedra products.

The study reviewed over sixteen thousand adverse events reported after ephedra use and found about twenty "sentinel events," including two deaths, four heart attacks, nine strokes, one seizure, and five psychiatric cases involving ephedra that occurred in the absence of other contributing factors. Now here's an important distinction in the RAND report—it called such cases "sentinel events," because they may indicate a safety problem but *do not prove that ephedra caused the adverse event.*

The HHS statement said the study "also found limited evidence of an effect of ephedra on short-term weight loss, and minimal evidence of an effect on performance enhancement in certain physical activities."

So there is no misunderstanding, I'm going to quote pertinent passages of the RAND study. Here is what it says:

Efficacy for Weight Loss

We identified 44 controlled trials that assessed use of ephedra or ephedrine used for weight loss. Of these, 18 were excluded from pooled analysis because they had a treatment duration of less than 8 weeks. Six additional trials were excluded for a variety of other reasons. Of the remaining 20 trials included in the meta-analysis, only five tested herbal ephedra-containing products.

Together, these 20 trials assessed 678 persons who consumed either ephedra or ephedrine. The majority of studies of both ephedra and ephedrine are plagued by methodological problems (particularly high attrition rates) that might contribute to bias. These methodological limitations must be considered when interpreting any conclusions regarding the efficacy of these products.

Nevertheless, the evidence we identified and assessed supports an association between short-term use of ephedrine, ephedrine plus caffeine, or dietary supplements that contain ephedra with or without herbs containing caffeine and a statistically significant increase in short-term weight loss (compared to placebo).

Adding caffeine to ephedrine modestly increases the amount of weight loss. There is no evidence that the effect of ephedra-containing dietary supplements with herbs containing caffeine differs from that of ephedrine plus caffeine: Both result in weight loss that is approximately 2 pounds per month greater than that with placebo, for up to 4 to 6 months. No studies have assessed the long-term effects of ephedra-containing dietary supplements or ephedrine on weight loss; the longest duration of treatment in a published study was 6 months.

Can you see the difference? As I've stated, HHS said the study "also found limited evidence of an effect of ephedra on short-term weight loss." But the actual report said, "Nevertheless, the evidence we identified and assessed supports an association between short-term use of ephedrine, ephedrine plus caffeine, or dietary supplements . . . *Both result in weight loss that is approximately 2 pounds per month greater than that with placebo, for up to 4 to 6 months*" (emphasis added).

When HHS states there is "limited evidence" of the herb's effectiveness for short-term weight loss and performance, do they mean more studies are needed or that the studies conducted so far haven't proved its effectiveness? After all, it doesn't say "showed limited or no effectiveness."

This is when I began to become suspicious.

Let's go to the next point, "Efficacy for Physical Performance Enhancement." The RAND researchers stated:

The effect of ephedrine on athletic performance was assessed in seven studies. No studies have assessed the effect of herbal ephedra-containing dietary supplements on athletic performance. The few studies that assessed the effect of ephedrine on athletic performance have, in general, included only small samples of fit individuals (young male military recruits) and have assessed the effects only on very short-term immediate performance. Thus, these studies did not assess ephedrine as it is used in the general population. The data support a modest effect of ephedrine plus caffeine on very short-term athletic performance. No studies have assessed the sustained use of ephedrine on performance over time. The only study that assessed the additive effects of these agents reported that ephedrine must be supplemented with caffeine to affect athletic performance.

Again, HHS said, ". . . and minimal evidence of an effect on performance enhancement in certain physical activities."

This made me perk up even more. While technically true, what the RAND researchers reported was it was difficult to evaluate because of a lack of data, *not* a lack of evidence supporting the contention that ephedra improved physical performance. A subtle difference in the use of words, but that subtle difference has enormous impact in what the words convey.

And it gets worse.

HHS also said the report concluded that "ephedra is associated with higher risks of mild to moderate side effects such as heart palpitations, psychiatric and upper gastrointestinal effects, and symptoms of autonomic hyperactivity such as tremor and insomnia, especially when it is taken with other stimulants."

HHS further states, "In conjunction with other recent studies of serious adverse events involving persons taking ephedra, the RAND study adds significantly to the evidence suggesting that ephedra as currently marketed may be associated with unreasonable safety risks."

Here's what RAND really stated:

The data on adverse events were drawn from clinical trials and case reports published in the literature, submitted to the FDA, and reported to Metabolife, a manufacturer of ephedra-containing supplement products. The strongest evidence for causality should come from clinical trials; however, in most circumstances, such trials do not enroll sufficient numbers of patients to adequately assess the possibility of rare outcomes. Such was the case with our review of ephedrine and ephedra-

What Is Meant by "Adverse Event"?

According to FDA regulations (21 CFR 312.32), a "serious adverse drug experience" with respect to human clinical experience includes "any experience that suggests a significant hazard, contraindication, side effect, or precaution." This includes "any experience that is fatal or life-threatening, is permanently disabling, requires inpatient hospitalization, or is a congenital anomaly, cancer, or overdose." Once an adverse event is reported it becomes an "AER."

In other words, If you take a product and develop a skin rash, that is an adverse event, but not necessarily a serious event. If you take a product and suffer a stroke as a result of a heart attack, that is a serious adverse event. If someone takes a drug or dietary supplement and dies from it, that is a very serious adverse event.

containing dietary supplements. Even in aggregate, the clinical trials enrolled only enough patients to detect a serious adverse event rate of at least 1.0 per 1,000.

For rare outcomes, we reviewed case reports, but a causal relationship between ephedra or ephedrine use and these events cannot be assumed or proven. Evidence from controlled trials was sufficient to conclude that the use of ephedrine and/or the use of ephedra-containing dietary supplements or ephedrine plus caffeine is associated with two to three times the risk of nausea, vomiting, psychiatric symptoms such as anxiety and change in mood, autonomic hyperactivity, and palpitations.

The majority of case reports are insufficiently documented to make an informed judgment about a relationship between the use of ephedrine or ephedra-containing dietary supplements and the adverse event in question.

For prior consumption of ephedra-containing products, we identified two deaths, three myocardial infarctions, nine cerebrovascular accidents, three seizures, and five psychiatric cases

EEC Expert Panel Consensus Statement

Available information does not demonstrate an association between the use of dietary supplements containing ephedrine alkaloids and serious adverse events when used according to industry recommendations for ephedra product. This recommendation includes 1) a serving limit of not more than 25 mg of total ephedrine alkaloids, 2) a limit on daily consumption of not more than 100 mg of total ephedrine alkaloids, and 3) appropriate warnings consistent with other available over-the-counter ephedrine alkaloid products.

All labeling of dietary supplements containing ephedrine alkaloids should contain appropriate directions and warnings for the public as adopted by the industry and similar to those approved for over-the-counter ephedrine alkaloid products.

The available information derived from studies of ephedrine and caffeine and dietary supplements containing ephedrine alkaloids supports the concept that dietary supplements containing ephedrine alkaloids may be useful in weight management.

Given the absence of data demonstrating an association between ephedra dietary supplements and serious adverse events, the presence or absence of a "susceptible population" cannot be determined. However, severe overdosing can lead to serious adverse events, and minor and/or very rare idiosyncratic reactions may occur (e.g., skin rashes, allergic reactions) with use at recommended serving sizes, as they can with any ingested food.

The pathology data available do not show any pattern consistent with ephedrine alkaloid-containing dietary supplements as a cause of death. An independent, multidisciplinary panel should be assembled to perform a clinical, pathological review of all deaths reported to FDA.

In order to provide a more comprehensive scientific database, the National Institutes of Health, Department of Health and Human Services, and industry should work together to consider further controlled studies to address unresolved issues.

Preparations that contain ephedrine alkaloids and are marketed without responsible label instructions and serving size limitations or are marketed with claims of achieving an altered state of consciousness or euphoria (including so called "street drug alternatives") should be prohibited because they promote excessive use and abuse.

More About the Ephedra Education Council Panel

Stephen E. Kimmel, M.D. Dr. Kimmel examined the appropriate scientific methods for assessing the safety of dietary supplements containing ephedra.

Stephen B. Karch, M.D. Dr. Karch reviewed the reports of serious cardiac events, and the published literature relevant to ephedra and its effects on the heart.

Norbert P. Page, M.S., D.V.M. Dr. Page is an expert in the preparation of toxicology profiles, toxicology testing, and compliance with regulatory requirements of the CPSC, EPA, OSHA, and FDA.

Theodore Farber, Ph.D., D.A.B.T. Since leaving government service and founding Toxichemica International with his partner, Dr. Norbert Page, Dr. Farber has served as an expert and lectured extensively on food, plant, drug toxicology, drug abuse, and risk assessment. Dr. Farber and Dr. Page assessed the causal relationship between ephedra and the new adverse event reports that the FDA released earlier this year and reviewed the published literature.

John W. Olney, M.D. He has conducted extensive research into the safety of food additives and dietary supplements, including monosodium glutamate (MSG) and aspartame.

Grover M. Hutchins, M.D. He conducted a comprehensive assessment of the serious cardiac events reported to the FDA as possibly associated with ephedra.

Edgar H. Adams, M.S., Sc.D. In 1999, he submitted testimony to FDA that there has been no evidence of significant abuse of ephedra products despite a long history of use. Dr. Adams has updated research on this issue.

as sentinel events; for prior consumption of ephedrine, we identified three deaths, two myocardial infarctions, two cerebrovascular accidents, one seizure, and three psychiatric cases as sentinel events. We identified 43 additional cases as possible sentinel events with prior ephedra consumption and seven additional cases as possible sentinel events for prior ephedrine consumption. About half the sentinel events occurred in persons aged 30 years or younger. Classification as a sentinel event does not imply a proven cause and effect relationship.

Did you notice of the sixteen thousand adverse events reported, only twenty instances caused alarm? Besides not flat-out blaming ephedra directly, the sentence by HHS that "ephedra as currently marketed may be associated with unreasonable safety risks," is also wide open to interpretation. It's not saying ephedra is dangerous, but rather that it could be a danger "as currently marketed." Can you see the distinction?

As for the future, here's what the RAND report recommended:

Future Research
Our analysis of the evidence reveals numerous gaps in the literature regarding the efficacy and safety of ephedra-containing dietary supplements. First, long-term assessments of the effectiveness of herbal ephedra or ephedrine for promoting weight loss are lacking. We identified no study with a treatment duration longer than 6 months. To improve health outcomes and reduce the risk of morbidities associated with being overweight, sufficient weight loss (5 to 10 percent of body weight) and long-term weight maintenance are necessary.

Therefore, the benefit of ephedrine or herbal ephedra-containing dietary supplements for health outcomes is unknown.

Evidence regarding the effect of herbal ephedra or ephedrine on physical performance that reflects its use in the general population (repeated or long-term use by a representative sample) is also needed.

In order to assess a causal relationship between ephedra or ephedrine consumption and serious adverse events, a hypothesis-testing study is needed.

Continued analysis of case reports cannot substitute for a properly designed study to assess causality. A case-control study would probably be the study design of choice.

I Am Not Making This Up

So, has the RAND report spurred the FDA to evaluate fairly whether ephedra is safe or effective? To the contrary—it has had the opposite effect.

Did HHS take the RAND report and say "we need to find out if ephedra provides long-term benefits by approving a large-scale study?"

No.

Did HHS take the RAND report and say "we need better studies?"

No.

Did HHS take the RAND report and say "we need to find out if the sentinel events imply a proven cause-and-effect relationship?"

Again, no.

Instead, HHS has stated that dietary supplements containing ephedra "may present significant or unreasonable risks as currently marketed," and announced a series of actions designed to protect Americans from these risks.

Besides the publication of the RAND study, what has happened to implement the recommendations from the Office of Women's Health, the Cantox Report and other studies in the last three years?

Virtually nothing. Nada. Zilch.

What the heck is going on here? In reality, a lot. As FDA Commissioner, Mark B. McClellan, M.D., Ph.D., stated in the

HHS press release, "The standard for regulating the safety of dietary supplements is largely untested, but we are committed to finding the right public health solution."

As you'll see in the following chapters, the FDA's interpretation of and response to the RAND report points to bigger issues than just the safety of ephedra. With the help of dramatic newspaper headlines after a couple of tragic incidents—dutifully reported by a compliant press—the next big meeting in July 2003 wasn't to gather information. It was more like a witch-hunt.

CHAPTER 5

The Case Against Ephedra

"I DROVE TO THE nearest gas station and purchased my own Yellow Jackets and Stackers. The label identified it as a diet supplement and high energizer containing twenty-five milligrams of ephedra and 300 milligrams of caffeine. Combine this with drinking Mountain Dew or Code Red and it would only enhance the caffeine level.

"Since the manufacturer's label stated that sales to a minor were prohibited, I asked the detectives if they would go to the distributors and request how they enforced sales. They discussed this first with the Logan County State Attorney's office and was informed that the warning was merely the manufacturer's and not a state law. He concluded that even a twelve-year-old could purchase them."

— Testimony of coroner Charles Fricke, Logan County, Illinois before the U.S. Senate Subcommittee on Oversight of Government Management, Restructuring, and the District of Columbia

Pushing for a Ban

It was a heartbreaking scene reported by television stations and newspapers across the country. On May 25, 2003, inside DePaul University's Athletic Center, Illinois Governor Rod Blagojevich signed into law a statewide ban on ephedra. "The FDA, I hope, will take notice of the fact that we, through the legislature and the governor signing a bill, have done what the FDA should have done a long time ago," said Governor Blagojevich. "And, hopefully, now they'll see a trend coming and they'll act to either regulate or, more importantly, ban the sale of ephedra."

Nearby were Debbie and Kevin Riggins, who had lost their son Sean, age sixteen, to a heart attack. They attribute his death to Yellow Jackets, an ephedra and caffeine product sold by New Jersey-based NVE Pharmaceuticals that Sean allegedly bought repeatedly. Yellow Jackets were displayed near the cash register at a local convenience store, undoubtedly near the chewing tobacco and steps away from the beer cooler. He and other athletes at his school were suspected of taking it for some time. While tobacco, alcohol and ephedra products all have warning labels, only the beer and tobacco are backed up by state law. Reports say store clerks seldom—if ever—checked the ages of the Yellow Jackets buyers.

The bill that Governor Blagojevich signed made it a misdemeanor to sell ephedra, punishable by up to a year in jail and a $5,000 fine. The measure passed both houses unanimously and the Illinois Retail Merchants Association has warned members to stop selling ephedra. The state plans to notify law enforcement agencies about the new law.

Mr. Riggins, who along with his wife pushed for the ban, also spoke. "I do have one message for the industry, and that is that ephedra's time is over. It is at an end," said Riggins, who has lobbied for the ban since his son died the previous fall, a day after playing middle linebacker for his Lincoln High School sophomore football team. For the Riggins family, the death toll from ephedra was 100 percent.

Governor Blagojevich urged other states and the federal government to adopt similar bans. "It's a good first step, but it's not enough." So far, New York and California are the only other states taking action. In May 2003, U.S. Senator Charles E. Schumer stood with members of the Westchester County Legislature and praised the legislature's plan to ban ephedra. That same month, the California State Senate approved a ban on ephedra-based products.

These weren't the only dramatic condemnations of ephedra. At the federal level, the House of Representatives held hearings in July 2003 and bills are pending in both the House and Senate that could do much more than ban or limit ephedra. Some members of Congress hope to alter—and possibly dismantle—the Dietary Supplement Health and Education Act (DSHEA) altogether, which, under a worst-case scenario, could make dietary supplements, including our daily vitamins, available only by prescription.

Piling On

Consumer watchdog groups have also joined the fray. On October 8, 2002, while giving testimony before the Senate Governmental Affairs Committee, Subcommittee on Oversight of Government Management Hearing on Dangers of Ephedra, the director of the Public Citizen Health Research Group, Sidney M. Wolfe, M.D., said the ephedra issue is not and has never been simply a question of scientific or medical evidence. Instead, he said, "It is a question of politics and the extraordinarily dangerous political cowardice of the FDA and HHS Secretary Thompson in the face of massive lobbying by ephedra-makers in Washington. Is the FDA still part of the Public Health Service or is it a drug-sales-promoting adjunct to the pharmaceutical and dietary supplements industries? De facto drug pushers include those who refuse to use their legal authority to remove a well-documented hazard to the public health from the market."

The following February, Bruce Silverglade, director of legal affairs for the Center for Science in the Public Interest (CSPI), said, "Ephedra has probably caused far more deaths and serious adverse reactions than any other dietary supplement on the market. If the FDA cannot restrict the sale of ephedra, there is little hope that it could protect consumers against other dietary supplements that pose substantial health risks." He added, "The FDA should ban the over-the-counter sale of ephedra, but as Secretary Thompson noted, the current law places a 'tough burden' on the government that prevents it from removing dangerous dietary supplements from the marketplace." Silverglade said it is up to Congress to enact legislation, "making it easier for the FDA to restrict the sales of ephedra and other herbal medicines that should not be used without a doctor's prescription."

While the concern of both these organizations is welcomed and to a degree, warranted, they are both off beam in certain critical areas. Simply put, the FDA possesses the authority to remove hazardous substances, and, as you'll see, the supplement industry has nowhere near the "buying power" of the pharmaceutical companies when it comes to lobbying or financial contributions to politicians.

League Limits

The United States Army and Air Force, the nation of Canada, the National Football League, Major League Soccer, Minor League Baseball, the National Collegiate Athletic Association (NCAA), and the International Olympic Committee have already outlawed the use of ephedra-based products. While

Major League Baseball hasn't banned it, many are calling for it to do so.

In 2002, Army and Air Force commissaries and post exchanges voluntarily removed all ephedra-containing dietary supplements from their shelves after the FDA received documentation regarding approximately 30 deaths between 1997 and 2001 of active duty personnel who were using these supplements—even though no direct cause-and-effect relation has been established. The Marines issued a similar ban in February 2001.

In June 2001, the Canadian government warned its citizens not to use these products, and in January 2002, it announced a recall of "ephedra/ephedrine products with labeled or implied claims for appetite suppression, weight loss promotion, metabolic enhancement, increased exercise tolerance, body-building effects, euphoria, increased energy or wakefulness, or other stimulant effects."

The NFL banned ephedra after the death of Minnesota Vikings offensive tackle Korey Stringer during training camp in 2001. A bottle of Ripped Fuel, which contains ephedra (and guarana, a source of caffeine), was found in Stringer's locker after he died, although Stringer's remains weren't tested for the substance—nor were any traces found inadvertently—during investigations of his death.

Fearful of legal repercussions, the NFL consulted with several experts and held a series of discussions and seminars about ephedra before training camp opened in 2002. The league banned all products containing the herbal stimulant ephedra or its alkaloids, and began random testing for it last summer after learning that dietary supplements supposedly increased the risk of heat-related illnesses. Players are tested and can be suspended after the first violation, as Carolina rookie Julius Peppers was for the final four games of last season. During 2003 training camps, the NFL suspended Minnesota Vikings tight end Byron Chamberlain for the first four games of the season for violating the league's policy on banned substances after he tested positive for ephedra. Chamberlain said he misread the label on a product he was using and believed it was ephedra-free.

Soon after, Denver Broncos safety Lee Flowers was suspended without pay for the first four games of the regular season for violating the NFL's banned substances policy. Flowers said he tested positive for ephedra but wasn't aware the supplement was in his system. He said his positive test stemmed from a vitamin he took in December.

In late July 2003, an attorney for Korey Stringer's widow said she was suing the NFL, alleging that the league's policies led to Stringer's heat-stroke-caused death during training camp in 2001. Stan Chesley said Kelci Stringer's suit would also name football helmet maker Riddell Sports Group Inc., and some NFL medical advisers. There was no mention of ephedra in the lawsuit.

Chesley said the federal lawsuit would include a wrongful death claim on behalf of Stringer's widow and son, and a class action claim on behalf of all NFL players. "What's on trial here is the rules and procedures and the culture" of the NFL, Chesley said. "Frankly, it's no coincidence that the average football player in the NFL plays for four and a half years. They use them up and spit them out."

Not all football players are happy about the ephedra punishments. Shortly after the ban, Philadelphia Eagles guard John Welbourn told *Sports Illustrated*, "The NFL basically scapegoated ephedra. The Chinese have been taking it for two thousand years. It's stupid. I worry a lot more about all the anti-inflammatories NFL teams hand out."

When reached for comment regarding the controversy, Rams running back Marshall Faulk also told *Sports Illustrated*, "They can ban it all they want, but I'm still going to take it."

Flowers, who appealed his suspension (but lost), also criticized the league's drug policy. "I would have been better off smoking crack. I would have got a slap on the wrist," Flowers said. "And that's a shame because here's something where we don't know what's going into these vitamins, but I can go out here and smoke crack and it's like, 'Well, you be careful next time.'"

Baseball Strikes Out on Ban

For Major League Baseball, the issue is much more complicated. According to an article posted on *PR Newswire* soon after Steve Bechler's death, Baltimore Orioles' owner Peter Angelos called upon Major League Baseball to ban ephedra. Critics say the Orioles organization tried to blame ephedra for Bechler's death, rather than allow the scrutiny that would surely come regarding the team's practices and policies during spring training workouts. One unnamed teammate said when Bechler reported to spring training out-of-shape that he was pushed extremely hard in the workouts. Twice, Orioles' manager Mike Hargrove pulled Bechler out of workouts and even considered a "special conditioning" program for the pitcher.

While the coroner who performed the autopsy on Bechler said ephedra probably contributed to his death, not everyone was so sure. Dr. Carlon M. Colker, a Greenwich, Connecticut physician, stated, "I don't see how ephedra could have contributed. This was clearly a case of heatstroke. Taking ephedra as directed does not lead to heatstroke."

On July 24, 2003, in front of the House Panel Hearing Testimony on Ephedra, Eugene Orza, associate general counsel of the Major League Baseball Players Association said "The position of the Players Association has long been that players should not be prohibited from using any substances that the United States government has effectively determined are not unsafe for consumption by other American consumers." Not quite a ringing endorsement, and probably more of a cop-out than anything. Still, many baseball players believe ephedra shouldn't be banned—possibly because many of them use it to endure a 162-game schedule, not to mention spring training and possible playoff games.

Orioles outfielder Jay Gibbons said he used ephedra in both college and pro ball. In the same *PR Newswire* piece mentioned above, he said, "It's a good supplement if taken right. I've never had any problems with it. I've never had any dizziness with it. It's just like caffeine." Gibbons indicated he used a supplement containing ephedrine to help drop about fifteen pounds before the 2002 season. This past winter, he did a better job of maintaining his weight, so he didn't need to use it. Gibbons' opinion is that using ephedrine is safe as long as people are careful to follow the labels.

Gibbons' teammate, David Segui added, "There's almost a witch-hunt going on" in the aftermath of Bechler's death. "It hasn't been proven that ephedrine caused his death. There was probably some milk found in his system, too. Did that cause his death?"

Orioles catcher Brook Fordyce said Steve Bechler's death probably wouldn't deter him from using ephedra. "It has no ill effect on me that I know of, and I use it safely. So if I was tired, I probably would take one, like if we had a day game after a night game. I'm not afraid of it."

Philadelphia Phillies rookie centerfielder Marlon Byrd said of ephedra, "It affects people differently, but no one should rush to conclusions."

Not everyone agrees. In May 2003, New York Mets catcher Mike Piazza said he stopped taking an ephedra-based supplement following Bechler's death. Piazza said he didn't use the supplement on a regular basis and quit completely after the Bechler incident. "I just used it a couple of times," Piazza said. "And this was before the guy (died). Obviously, I wouldn't recommend it now."

Piazza was prompted to talk about the issue after a story ran in *Playboy* magazine that quoted the star catcher as saying, "Ripped Fuel is kind of cool." As I mentioned previously,

Ripped Fuel is the ephedra supplement found in the locker of Minnesota Vikings player Korey Stringer.

It's probably important to note that the *PR Newswire* article (in which Orioles owner Peter Angelos called for a ban on ephedra and which quotes several baseball players) originated with Cytodyne Technologies—which recently changed its name to Nutraquest Inc.—the maker of the ephedra product that Steve Bechler consumed.

Pharmacists and the AMA Prescribe Ban

The American Society of Health-System Pharmacists (ASHP) has urged the FDA to ban the sale of dietary supplements containing ephedra. The ASHP said labeling changes proposed by the FDA will not protect the public from the dangers of these products.

In its letter to the FDA on April 4, 2003, ASHP stated it supported a ban on ephedra products because it is convinced ephedrine alkaloids pose a significant risk of illness and injury. "Using these products represents significant expenditures for a remedy of unsubstantiated value; and other safe and effective interventions are available for all common uses of these products."

ASHP also encouraged the agency to work with Congress to amend the Dietary Supplement Health Education Act (DSHEA) to require that dietary supplements must at least meet the same legal requirements as nonprescription drugs. It's easy to see where ASHP's interests lie—in filling prescriptions of pharmaceutical drugs, or at least guaranteeing the purchase of OTC medications.

That's why it is not surprising that ASHP is adamantly opposed to legislation passed at the end of July 2003 by the U.S. House of Representatives allowing medications to freely move across U.S. borders without authorization or control by the FDA. "This bill is absolutely the wrong way to solve the important issue of medication affordability and accessibility in the

U.S.," said Henri R. Manasse, Jr., Ph.D., Sc.D., ASHP executive vice president and CEO. "Allowing imported drugs to enter the country with the bare minimum in terms of safeguards will create significant safety hazards for patients who cannot know if the medications they are receiving are expired, contaminated, counterfeit, subpotent, or superpotent."

Known as "reimportation," the law allows Americans to purchase the drugs, which were originally manufactured in the United States, from foreign suppliers at the cheaper prices.

The House legislation allows only for importation of drugs approved by the FDA and calls for protective packaging to ensure safety. However, many of these drugs are actually made in the United States. Countries such as Canada have government-imposed price controls, so U.S. companies sell their products for less there than they do in the United States.

At a press conference in the Capitol, Senator Debbie Stabenow of Michigan demonstrated two protective technologies that she said could prevent counterfeiting. One—color-shifting dyes that change color when viewed at different angles—already is used on new $20 bills (and will be used with other currencies) as well as on vials of some HIV-AIDS medications. The other protection is a computer chip currently used by Wal-Mart that prevents any tampering with sealed packaging. By utilizing this readily available technology and allowing imports from the twenty-five countries included in the House bill, she said, "We could right now cut drug prices literally in half." Stabenow said she knows the fight will be difficult since there are six drug industry lobbyists for every senator.

"Big pharma" (as it's often referred to in industry and political circles) has another powerful friend, the American Medical Association (AMA), who also wants to do away with ephedra. It's no secret many physicians feel threatened by dietary supplements. They see many of the claims as "hype" and worry about patients using unproven products in lieu of traditional medical treatments. From the outset, it was the clear intent of Congress in enacting DSHEA that consumers should be provided with products, information and education that would help promote health and prevent disease. Yet, since Congress noted in its "findings" section of the Act that "consumers should be empowered to make choices about preventive health care programs based on data from scientific studies of health benefits related to particular dietary supplements," the AMA has balked.

When testifying before the Subcommittee on Oversight of Government Management, Restructuring and the District of Columbia on October 8, 2002, Ron Davis, M.D., a member of the Board of Trustees of the AMA, stated, "The AMA recognizes that it is difficult to prove cause-and-effect relationships based on voluntary AERs. Nonetheless, the primary question that should be considered by the FDA is whether manufacturers' claims of purported benefits for these products outweigh the products' risks. We continue to believe that the benefits do not outweigh the risks, and the weight of the available clinical evidence supports the removal of dietary supplement products containing ephedrine alkaloids from the market."

The AMA carries a great deal of weight and their concerns and opinions are taken very seriously. However, Dr. Davis also said the following, "Because dietary supplements are classified as foods rather than drugs, rigorous safety and efficacy standards are not required for these products."

Huh? This statement is absolutely false, and Dr. Davis should know better. When the Dietary Supplement Health and Education Act (DSHEA) of 1994 was enacted, it established dietary supplements as a new category distinct from both foods and drugs with separate regulations for that category.

Although I've already defined what a dietary supplement is according to the FDA, it is important enough to once again repeat. According to DSHEA, a dietary supplement is:

• A product, other than tobacco, which is used in conjunction with a healthy diet and contains one or more of the following dietary ingredients: a vitamin, mineral, herb or other botanical, an amino acid, a dietary substance for use by man to supplement the diet by increasing the total daily intake, or a concentrate, metabolite, constituent, extract, or combinations of these ingredients

- Intended for ingestion in pill, capsule, tablet or liquid form
- Not represented for use as a conventional food or as the sole item of a meal or diet
- Labeled as a "dietary supplement"

This includes products such as an approved new drug, certified antibiotic, or licensed biologic that was marketed as a dietary supplement or food before approval, certification, or license (unless the Secretary of Health and Human Services waives this provision).

Clearly, supplements are *not* classified as a food and regulated as such.

Dissent, Anyone?

Just because the AMA released an official statement on behalf of its members doesn't mean that all its members agree with it. In a letter to Health and Human Services Secretary Tommy Thompson in January 2003, more than twenty board-certified physicians stated their support of ephedra dietary supplements. The physicians cited their patients' struggles with obesity and their need for continued access to safe and beneficial ephedra products.

The letter urges continued availability of the products, but with appropriate label instructions. The letter recognizes some of the problems faced by the HHS and FDA. "I applaud your efforts to prevent marketers from advertising and selling illegal and harmful ephedra products, such as Yellow Jacket and herbal XTC, as alternatives to street drugs." While twenty doctors out of the vast AMA membership might not seem like much, the point is there are doctors who believe the AMA is not speaking for them. Are they the recipients of under-the-table payments from dietary supplement companies? I honestly don't know. If so, it would probably have to be a heck of a lot of money for them to stake their reputations on such a controversial issue.

Mass Media or Mass Hysteria?

The FDA, other state and federal regulatory agencies and other organizations frequently issue press releases concerning ephedra supplements and drug products containing the pure alkaloid ephedrine. More often than not, they claim the products are associated with numerous AERs. Reporters faced with tight deadlines are sometimes forced to resort to these press releases churned out by government agencies and other organizations for background material on complicated issues.

This certainly is true when the subject is ephedra. As a result, these products are almost always reported in the popular press as potentially unsafe. That's why it's easy to find the same statements repeated over and over and over. As you know, the more something is said over and over, the more likely it will eventually be accepted as truth.

Believe it or not, sometimes these organizations get it wrong. Here's a perfect example. On February 28, 2003, a Consumer Advisory on ephedra was distributed by the National Center for Complementary and Alternative Medicine (NCCAM), which is part of the National Institutes of Health. The first line of the advisory reads, "Dietary supplements containing ephedra, which have been in the news recently because of the deaths of well-known athletes, may cause rare but serious health consequences" (see Figure 1 on opposite page).

Which "well-known athletes"? Sean Riggins, the high school player in Illinois? Steve Bechler, who wasn't sure he would even

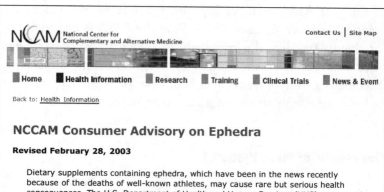

Figure 1. Portion of page on NCCAM's website listing its advisory on ephedra
(http://nccam.nih.gov/health/alerts/ephedra/consumeradvisory.htm)

make the Orioles team? Neither of them fit the description "well-known (unless, of course, you count the publicity they received *after* they died). Korey Stringer? He had an ephedra product in his locker, but there is no evidence that he took it. Are we now supposed to assume that he did simply to help build more evidence for the case against ephedra?

Consider how the issue is covered in a May 1, 2003 *Sports Illustrated* article entitled, "NFL puts support behind supplement regulation laws." The article states, "The NFL banned ephedra after the death of Minnesota Vikings offensive tackle Korey Stringer during training camp in 2001 . . ." Doesn't that imply he died from ephedra? Shouldn't there be a caveat such as "although there is no evidence he ever took it"? By not including a clarifying statement, the sentence very much implies that ephedra caused Stringer's death. Even those who know better might conclude that new evidence surfaced without them knowing it.

Then there's the strange case of Rashidi Wheeler, a football player at Northwestern University. Wheeler collapsed and died on Aug. 3, 2001, after participating in a conditioning drill. His parents sued Northwestern, claiming officials did not give their son proper medical treatment. Northwestern argued that ephedra-containing supplements Wheeler was taking caused his death.

The filing came a few days after attorneys for Wheeler's mother, Linda Will, accused the school of a cover-up after discovering a university doctor had destroyed records of a physical he performed on Wheeler weeks before the football player's death. In November 2001, Will's lawyers submitted a list of the contents in Wheeler's locker that did not mention any dietary supplements containing ephedra.

According to the Associated Press, James Montgomery, an attorney for Will, said Northwestern representatives were present when Wheeler's family cleaned out his locker. "There was no ephedra in there," Montgomery said. "There was none of the other stuff that they said was in there that contained ephedra."

So who are the "well-known athletes" NCCAM had in mind when it wrote its "Consumer Advisory"? I don't have a clue, but you can bet the statement is now widely accepted as fact. Once a barn door is opened . . .

Side Effects: Ephedra vs. Pharmaceuticals

In the last chapter I discussed the findings of the seven scientists who, in August 2000, appeared at the Office of Women's Health at the Department of Health and Human Services for two days of hearings about the safety of ephedra. You heard or read about these findings didn't you? What—you didn't hear about them? No surprise there, I suppose—the hearings garnered little publicity.

There's a greater chance you read this story, which appeared in *USA Today* on July 17, 2003. Here's the headline: "As Backlash Against Ephedra Mounts, Congress Drags Feet."

There was a three-year gap between the panel's findings and the *USA Today* story. Much had to have changed in that time, right? More evidence of ephedra's dangers, a higher percentage of adverse side effects and many more deaths from its use, wouldn't you think? Well, let's see:

- Baseball player Steve Bechler died.
- High school football player Sean Riggins died.
- Korey Stringer had an ephedra product in his locker.

Now let's look at some other statistics. Over those same three years, it's estimated that:

- 300 people died as a result of using acetaminophen.
- Thousands of people died due to the misuse of aspirin (some studies place the number as high as 48,000).
- 137,000 people die each year just as a result of taking prescription medications where no prescription errors or abuse are involved.
- 300,000 died from alcohol use.*
- 1,300,000 died from cigarette use.*

(*These are not regulated by FDA)

Now look at the data from the 2001 National Household Survey on Drug Abuse, SAMHSA, 2002 regarding Emergency Department Trends from the Drug Abuse Warning Network. In 2000, 43 percent of those who ended up in hospital emergency rooms from drug overdoses—*nearly a half million people*—were there because of misusing prescription drugs. Not illicit drugs, but perfectly legal prescription drugs.

In seven cities in 2000 (Atlanta, Chicago, Los Angeles, Miami,

New York, Seattle, and Washington, D.C.), 626 people died from overdose of painkillers and tranquilizers. By 2001, such deaths had increased in Miami and Chicago by 20 percent. From 1998 to 2000, the number of people entering an emergency room because of misusing hydrocodone (Vicodin) rose 48 percent, oxycodone (OxyContin) 108 percent, and methadone 63 percent. The rates are intensifying: from mid-2000 to mid-2001, oxycodone misuse went up 44 percent in emergency room visits.

By comparison the highest number of deaths attributed to ephedra is 130—and that's for the herb's roughly decade-long use as a weight-loss and fitness aid. (Although I've seen this number stated a few times, I have no idea where it originated.) But even that number is highly questionable. According to the RAND study, there were only seventeen "sentinel" events where death was only one outcome. And even these deaths, since they are based on AER data, could be wrong. Some experts put the number of deaths where there is no question that ephedra was the culprit at only two. Yet here's a sample of media reports reporting the number of ephedra deaths:

October 8, 2002 Associated Press
"FDA Cracks Down On Illegally Promoted Ephedra Product"
" . . . said Sen. Dick Durbin, an Illinois Democrat. He said Food and Drug Administration reports link ephedra to eighty-one deaths and 1,400 incidents of heart attack, high blood pressure and stroke."

February 26, 2003 *Sports Illustrated*
"Why the Federal Govt. Needs to Come to Terms with Ephedra"
"But Bechler didn't listen, and he joins a grim roll of nearly 90 deaths . . ."

May 16, 2003 *State Journal-Register* (IL)
"Ephedra-based products have been blamed for dozens of deaths, including that of 16-year-old Lincoln Community High

Adverse Events Associated with Ephedra and Ephedrine, as Described in the RAND Report

Event	Number of Events	Number of Sentinel Events	Number of Possible Sentinel Events
Death	84	5	12
Myocardial Infarction (heart attack)	26	5	7
Other Cardiac	30	0	3
Cerebrovascular Event (stroke)	56	11	12
Seizure	40	4	7
Other Neurological	8	0	1
Psychiatric Event	91	8	8

School football player Sean Riggins, who took it along with caffeinated soda, believing his athletic performance would be enhanced."

May 25, 2003 *State of Illinois News page*
Office of the Governor:
" . . . ephedra—the controversial herbal weight-loss, body-building and athletic enhancing supplement that has been linked to more than one hundred deaths and 18,000 other medical problems—and he called on other states to follow suit."

May 26, 2003 *San Diego Union-Tribune*
"Ephedra, blamed for nearly 120 deaths, drew national attention after officials investigating the February heatstroke death of Baltimore Orioles pitching prospect Steve Bechler linked it to a diet pill containing ephedrine, ephedra's active ingredient.

Although the number seems to climb by date, that is merely a coincidence. *If* there were that many new deaths, you would have heard the specifics. In fact, it would have been unavoidable.

We Report, *We* (Not You) Decide

Let's look a little closer at the July 17 *USA Today* story, which by the way, has no byline:

"Years after diet supplements containing ephedra surged onto store shelves without government regulation or consumer warnings, concerns about serious risks to users finally are forcing meaningful changes. On Monday, New Jersey's attorney general joined a parade of more than one hundred lawsuits against the ephedra industry."

Actually, there *is* government regulation—the DSHEA, for one, as well as the power of the FDA to remove any product it deems dangerous. And there have been consumer warnings. His mention of "meaningful changes" is correct; especially if the author is referring to the changes in labeling. However, that doesn't quite jive with the next sentence about the lawsuits. Sorry if I seem picky, but did the lawsuits bring about the "meaningful changes"? Or did the author add that sentence simply for dramatic affect?

The next paragraph states, "The popular herbal supplement, which is linked to at least 120 deaths and 1,400 serious reactions, also is under assault from state legislatures, medical groups—and the marketplace. Last week, CVS, the nation's second-largest drugstore chain, announced it will stop selling ephedra diet products."

The article is 100 percent correct about CVS actions. But what it fails to report is that when CVS announced it would stop selling ephedra-based products it also stated its belief that ephedra-based products are safe when used as directed. This is similar to a statement made by the largest American vitamin and dietary supplement chain, General Nutrition Centers (GNC), in May when it announced it would stop selling the herb. Here are the exact words from the GNC release dated May 2, 2003, "We believe that ephedra-based products are safe when used as directed. Nonetheless, the current business climate dictates that we move in a different direction," said Michael K. Meyers, GNC's president and CEO.

Could it be both chains are simply responding to a lessening demand for the products? Are they afraid of liability for future and past sales of ephedra? Probably so, especially considering the phrase "the current business climate dictates that we move in a different direction" in GNC's press release. It's also interesting that CVS will still gladly sell you prescription drugs, OTC pain relievers, and in most locations, cigarettes.

Later in the USA Today article, the author writes: "Congress continues to protect the diet supplements industry, the source of $4 million in political contributions during the past six years."

I have heard this charge many times. If I didn't know better, I'd be incensed. Four million dollars in campaign contributions over the past six years? Those scallywags! But wait—while $4 million is certainly a lot of money, according to the Center for Responsive Politics the total amount of political contributions from dietary supplement companies in the 2002 election cycle was $969,642 with the large majority of it—$847,750—coming from one company, Metabolife. During the same period, the pharmaceutical companies gave $26.9 million. Yes, you read that right—$26.9 million.

This is probably a good time to talk a little about Metabolife. On August 15, 2002, the Justice Department launched a criminal investigation of Metabolife to determine whether the herbal diet pill manufacturer lied about ephedra's safety. The next day, Metabolife, with estimated annual sales of $500 million, produced thirteen thousand consumer complaints about ephedra products. The company said that these health-related complaints were not released because they hadn't been analyzed properly. The explanation angered U.S. Food and Drug Administration officials, who have sought access to the documents since 1997. Calling it "disingenuous," FDA Deputy Commissioners Lester Crawford declared that "Metabolife has refused and resisted us every step of the way."

Back to the *USA Today* story, which continues, "While a House subcommittee resumes desultory hearings next week on the supplement's dangers, there's little movement toward what's really needed: government regulation of ephedra and other largely untested and unproved diet supplements."

Not so. Pending before the U.S. Senate is the proposed legislation S.722 ("Dietary Supplement Safety Act of 2003"), which could be voted on at any time (possibly before you read this book). Just in case you were wondering, this could be the first step toward the dismantling of the DSHEA codes, ultimately affecting how your supplements are regulated, their cost, and their availability.

The article continues, "The RAND Corp. think tank issued a review in February concluding that while several instances of death and illness are clearly linked to ephedra use, the product does not result in long-term weight-loss benefits or improvements in athletic performance."

In case you missed it, I covered the RAND report in Chapter 4. It says nothing of the sort. This is what it says: "No studies have assessed the long-term effects of ephedra-containing dietary supplements or ephedrine on weight loss; the longest duration of treatment in a published study was six months." Folks, that's a big difference between the two statements.

Going on with the *USA Today* article: "The industry defends its product by attacking studies as inconclusive and quoting the odd positive line from largely negative conclusions."

Seems that this author is guilty of doing exactly what he's criticizing.

Let's consider some additional statements from the *USA Today* article: "Two major ephedra producers based in Florida and Arizona agreed July 1 to repay customers $370,000 to resolve deceptive-advertising charges," and

"A California judge issued a $12.5 million false-advertising judgment last month against the maker of the weight-loss pill implicated in the death of a Baltimore Orioles pitcher this year."

As well they should. It is against the law—including DSHEA—to run false advertising. No one except the guilty parties have defended this behavior.

Here's another: "The judge also found that the firm had pressured its researchers into bending their reports to be more favorable."

Is this true? To some extent. Now I know *USA Today* specializes in tight, concise stories, but this line just dangles there and is open to any sort of speculation. Here's a different account, which appears in the June 23, 2003 *New York Times* about evidence that surfaced during the false-advertising trial in California against Cytodyne Technologies, maker of Xenadrine RFA-1, the supplement implicated in the death of Steve Bechler. Written by Ford Fessenden, the *Times* article illustrates how the company tried to influence one researcher. The researcher, Jeffrey Armstrong of Eastern Michigan University, had refused to rewrite a journal abstract the way the company wanted, according to testimony, and Tim Ziegenfuss, the consultant who commissioned the study on behalf of the company, said he would try to change Dr. Armstrong's mind.

"As far as rewriting the abstract, since I am not recognized as a co-author on the study I am not allowed to do it," Dr. Ziegenfuss said on November 2000 in an e-mail message to a company official. He added, "In this case the best I can do is try to carefully nudge his interpretation/writing in Cytodyne's favor."

Cytodyne was unable to budge Dr. Armstrong: "I will not be intimidated," he said in an e-mail message after being told that the company was threatening to sue him. But in another message, Dr. Ziegenfuss suggested that the study could still be marketed.

"Let Jeff do his hum-drum 'science' thing," he said. "This

will portray Cytodyne in an objective, favorable manner to the scientific community," he added. "This is particularly important now, considering the recent bad press on ephedrine. And then since Jeff has no control over the use of data in ads, use percentage changes there to impress consumers." The company did, turning a modest 3.1-pound average weight loss over several weeks into exclamatory copy.

It seems that Cytodine tried to pressure the researcher, but failed. Good for the researcher. And let's not kid ourselves. Anyone who thinks this type of behavior is limited to dietary supplement companies is naïve. Sadly, this behavior is widespread, used to promote numerous products ranging from baby cribs to foods to pharmaceutical drugs. As for false advertising claims, only someone who never watches TV or reads newspapers and magazines would believe the practice isn't commonplace.

While this justification doesn't make the tactic acceptable, it does make one wonder why ephedra is singled out to be the focus of so much negative press.

Back to the *USA Today* article:

> Such actions have made an impact. Sales surveys indicate business is off 30 percent or more for some of the most popular ephedra potions. But scattershot court rulings and state laws can't provide the seamless national protection the public needs.
>
> The FDA now is asking for more evidence about ephedra's health risks, and it is considering some halfway protections, including warning labels and added actions to discourage exaggerated marketing claims.
>
> The better answer is Congressional action giving the FDA the same power to regulate supplements as it does similarly dangerous drugs. Instead, Congress gave the industry a generous immunity from regulation nine years ago and has stubbornly refused to reconsider the issue ever since.
>
> Until that changes, the public is left to look elsewhere for whatever spotty protection it can get.

Again this is patently untrue. There is no "generous immunity," as I've already explained in Chapter 3. The simple truth is, the FDA can and does regulate ephedra—and it can take ephedra off the market if it proves it is dangerous. But they haven't, whatever the reasons. If this isn't part of a larger plan to destroy DSHEA—which reporters might be promoting without being fully aware of the facts—I don't know what is.

More Bad Reporting

Consider another story, this time appearing on MSNBC in April 2001. Entitled "Unsafe Supplements?" it is almost entirely inaccurate and misleading. I've already covered many of the issues that correspondent Robert Hager raises, so I'll only discuss other issues.

First of all, the theme of the report is that public health is being endangered by the lack of oversight in the diet supplement industry, and that new government regulation is needed. As I've said repeatedly—and will say again—the FDA already has the authority to remove dangerous products from the marketplace.

In writing about the dangers of supplements, the media fails to compare the pharmaceutical industry—which is highly regulated and has plenty of government oversight—and the amount of deaths due to its products, namely prescription and OTC drugs.

I think we need to follow the money. What health and safety worries does the NIH *really* have about dietary supplements if, according to government figures, it allocates a mere 1 percent of the amount expended annually for medical and health research to supplements? That's right—1 percent! If it really were concerned about establishing, through legitimate research, the safety and/or dangers of ephedra and other supplements, wouldn't it dedicate more of its funds to that endeavor?

The MSNBC story stated the FDA is often not informed of adverse reactions. "The government doesn't hear about the vast majority of health problems associated with dietary supplements, according to an unpublished report from the inspector general of the Department of Health and Human Services."

The story talks about one particular problem; that state Poison Control Centers aren't communicating with the FDA. While this may be true, wouldn't this be the case with any substance people take, not just supplements? And wouldn't these communications channels be easily established if there was sufficient data to warrant such an action?

The MSNBC story also states that the FDA "was unable to determine the ingredients in 32 percent of the products mentioned in adverse event reports." According to the FDA's own regulation, as of March 23, 1999 dietary supplement products must include an ingredient statement and information panel titled "Supplement Facts," in which all ingredients in the product must be declared.

The MSNBC story goes on to say "in a recent year when the FDA received 470 reports of bad reactions to dietary supplements, the nation's poison control clinics actually treated 13,000." First, just as we indicated in the discussion about AERs (adverse event reports), it is impossible to determine if these cases can be directly attributed to dietary supplements, whether they were only a contributing factor, or if the supplements were merely present in the victims' stomachs. We also don't know whether they were due to a deliberate overdose, an accidental overdose or people not following directions on the label. But even if they do point to supplements as the culprits, this means that thirteen thousand reports of adverse reactions represent *less than one-hundredth of one percent* of the 150 million Americans taking supplements, or approximately one person out of 11,536.

The article then mentions the ephedra uproar. The MSNBC story states "Research on ephedra that was commissioned by the FDA concluded that the supplement poses risks that far outweigh any benefits it might have. Results were published in the *New England Journal of Medicine*."

There are a couple problems with this. First, this *NEJM* article was not new. Second, it certainly was *not* clinical research. Rather, it was a study of anecdotal reports collected by the FDA. Anecdotal reports don't constitute unbiased research, nor do all experts agree with the conclusions in the *NEJM* article.

One of the EEC's panel of seven, Dr. Grover M. Hutchins, conducted his own analysis of twenty-two reports from the same FDA data in which death occurred. In a letter to the *NEJM*, Dr. Hutchins stated that the data "showed no consistent clinical or pathological features of the reported adverse events and showed that ephedrine-type alkaloids were not likely to have been causative or contributing factors in the deaths. . . . With an adequate explanation of the reported adverse events, the implication of ephedrine-type alkaloids in deaths from a wide variety of conditions that occur in the general population is no more than idle speculation."

Bruce Silverglade from the Center for Science in the Public Interest is also quoted in the article. He said, "Right now consumers are playing a game of Russian roulette because no one is sorting out products that work from those that don't." His statement is not entirely true.

Reputable supplement manufacturers do conduct efficacy research. Also, two agencies in the federal Department of Health and Human Services (HHS)—the Office of Dietary Supplements and the National Center for Complementary and Alternative Medicine—are funding efficacy research. Additionally, the Office of Dietary Supplements has created a database of research about dietary supplements—IBIDS—which now contains nearly half-a-million bibliographic records about dietary supplements from 1986 to the present.

As for product testing to find out which supplements "work," the website ConsumerLab.com compares products with formulations shown to be effective in clinical trials. Finally, other organizations are developing third-party testing and certification programs.

Boozer Under Attack

Next, the MSBNC story saw fit to take a swipe at the research by Dr. Carol Boozer, which I described in the last chapter, by stating "While the FDA has received claims of 70 deaths among ephedra users, an industry-financed study turned up no problems."

In describing Dr. Boozer's research as "industry-financed," MSNBC implies it was automatically biased and therefore, crooked. Most research on drugs is at least partially financed by the pharmaceutical companies. (I cover a number of medical conferences, so I know.)

Actually, while the FDA "study" was no study at all, but rather a review of unproven anecdotal cases, Boozer's study used "the gold standard" of research: a randomized, double-blind, placebo-controlled clinical trial. Isn't this what everyone wants?

While Metabolife contributed their product and some funding to Dr. Boozer's study, the funding was indirect; the money went through Science Toxicology and Technology, an independent consulting firm of physicians and toxicologists based in San Francisco that underwrote the research.

While accurately quoting Dr. Boozer as saying, "The bottom line is that in our studies we found that there were no real health consequences, significant health consequences, to individuals that were taking these products," it said she was affiliated with the New York Obesity Research Center. For the average person, this would mean nothing. The story neglects to mention that the New York Obesity Research Center is affiliated with the prestigious Columbia Medical School.

Dr. Boozer did manage to make an excellent point in the MSNBC article. Referring to the *NEJM* article mentioned above, Boozer noted twelve million people took ephedra in 1999. She pointed out that whenever twelve million people do the same thing—such as get haircuts, drink water, take aspirin, or drive to work—some will have heart attacks, develop high blood pressure, or suffer strokes—and some will die either because of or in spite of their activities. (As you'll see later, the ephedra enemies weren't done with Dr. Boozer.)

As its final point, the MSNBC story lists three recommendations from the report given by the inspector general of the Department of Health and Human Services. One of those recommendations is that "ingredients in supplements should be standardized to guard against contamination." That's misleading. Contamination is largely caused by poor manufacturing practices—things like incomplete cleaning of machines—and not raw materials. For eight years—since DSHEA went into effect—the FDA has promised to develop "good manufacturing practice" (GMP) standards that all supplement manufacturers will be required to meet. The National Nutritional Foods Association (NNFA) already has a GMP inspection and certification program in place, complete with a seal that companies can place on their labels.

Even without a GMP, dietary supplements are already required to be both safe and pure (free of pathogenic contaminants) under the FDA's current GMP standards for foods, which supplements can be held to as a fall back position. The FDA's new GMP standards for dietary supplements are expected to be tougher than those for foods largely because the procedures for processing supplements are more complex and in some ways more technically challenging than those for foods.

Money, Money, Money

At this point you might be asking yourself why the dietary supplement industry is characterized by so many as an out-of-control, undependable trade run by a scurrilous lot of incompetents and crooks. Well, those are especially strong words so let me rephrase the question—why are so many people out to hinder, if not destroy, the dietary supplement industry?

I think it's obvious there are those in and out of the HHS and FDA who have objected to DSHEA since it's inception as just a bad law, and who have used ephedra as the "poster child" of their objections. Of course, the cynic in me believes it has to do more with what is so often the root of much disagreement today—that's right, money. For example, one company making ephedra-caffeine products reportedly grossed $946 million yearly during its peak. If you consider the growth of the supplement industry into a $4-billion-a-year industry since DSHEA passed in 1994, well, it's not hard to believe that there parties outside the industry that desire a piece of the pie.

Although not many people are anxious to speak on the record about whom they think is really pushing for a ban on ephedra and overhauling DSHEA, at least one man is. "The pharmaceutical industries have huge political lobbies," said Richard B. Kreider, Ph.D., Professor & Chair of the Exercise & Sport Nutrition Laboratory, Center for Exercise, Nutrition & Preventive Health Research at Baylor University. Dr. Kreider, who is also president of the American Society of Exercise Physiologists, also pointed out that Dr. Frank Greenway, one of the EEC Seven and an internationally recognized expert in bariatric medicine from the Pennington Biomedical Research Center, reported that ephedra worked as well and was more cost effective than several diet drugs, which must have at least some pharmaceutical companies nervous. "The pharmaceutical lobby also has an interest to see supplements that may work as well as some (other) drugs be restricted."

Could Dr. Kreider be right? This is a good time to take a closer look.

CHAPTER 6

The Name-and PR-Game

WE'VE ALL HEARD IT BEFORE. A news anchor says or a magazine writer states, "According to experts . . ." And it's so common, we don't even think about it. And we also assume that whoever this "expert" may be—a professor, doctor or watchdog group spokesperson—must be on the level. But how do we really know? How often is it revealed who those experts are, where they get their funding, or with what organization(s) they're associated?

There are trade groups and lobbyists for every imaginable commodity. The beef, sugar, dairy—and yes, the dietary supplement—industries, including one for ephedra, all have organizations whose primary (or sole) function is to trumpet how wonderful their products are and beat back and diminish any criticism.

Other organizations within the public relations industry also do a lot of product pushing for certain companies and industries, but you'd never know it from their names. The public relations industry has spent years and millions of dollars funding and creating industry front groups posing as dispensers of "sound" science. In reality, their "sound science" is simply product spin defined by the drug, tobacco, chemical, genetic engineering, petroleum and other industries.

Here are examples of such "front" groups:

- *American Council on Science and Health (ACSH):* Receives financial support from about three hundred different sources, including foundations, trade associations, corporations and individuals.
- *Center for Consumer Freedom (CCF):* A front group for the tobacco, restaurant and liquor industries that represents itself as an advocate for consumers' rights.
- *Consumer Alert:* Funded by corporations, CA opposes flame-resistance standards for clothing fabrics issued by the Consumer Product Safety Commission, and defends products such as the diet drug dexfenfluramine (Redux), which was taken off the market because of its association with heart valve damage. In contrast with Consumers Union, which is funded primarily by member subscriptions, Consumer Alert is funded by the industries whose products it defends—companies like Pfizer Pharmaceuticals, Philip Morris, Eli Lilly, Monsanto, Upjohn, Chemical Manufacturers Association, Ciba-Geigy, the Beer Institute, Coors and Chevron USA.
- *International Food Information Council Foundation (IFIC):* IFIC—which receives its financial support from the food, beverage and agricultural industries—says the mission of its foundation is to convey science-based information on food safety and nutrition to consumers, health professionals, educators, journalists and government officials. While IFIC says its goal is to bridge the informational gap by collecting and disseminating scientific information, what IFIC fails to reveal are the names of the companies that finance it. It's an impressive list and includes Coca-Cola, Pepsi, Hershey, M&M/Mars Candy, and Procter & Gamble.

All these groups (and there are many, many others) support

research and trumpet results favorable to their clients and those who finance their operations. What kind of findings do you think they would support? Those disparaging what they sell?

Quietly financed by the industries whose products they—ahem—evaluate, these "independent" research agencies churn out "scientific" studies and press materials announcing "breakthrough" research to every radio station and newspaper in the country, endeavoring to create the image their underwriters want.

Many of these carefully scripted reports are molded in a news format and can be read like straight news. This saves journalists the trouble of researching the subjects on their own, especially on topics about which they know very little. Entire sections of the release can be used intact with no editing, given the byline of the reporter or newspaper or TV station.

Does this really happen? According to research by the Center for Media & Democracy (CMD), a nonprofit, public-interest organization that conducts investigative reports on the public relations industry, sometimes as many as half the stories appearing in an issue of the *Wall Street Journal* are based solely on such press releases. These types of stories are mixed right in with legitimately researched stories. Unless you have done the research yourself, it's nearly impossible to tell the difference.

"Ask Your Doctor About . . ."

The global pharmaceutical industry—which generated revenues of more than $364 billion in 2001—is the world's most profitable stock market sector. According to IMS Health, the leading drug industry market analyst, half the global drug sales are in the U.S. alone, with Europe and Japan accounting for another 37 percent.

While the pharmaceutical industry likes to foster the impression that it is weighed down by research and development expense, the reality is that public relations, marketing and administration commonly absorb twice the amount spent on the research and development of drugs. During 2000 more than $13.2 billion was spent on pharmaceutical marketing in the U.S. alone. (We'll discuss this more in a later chapter.)

Advancing the pharmaceutical industry's case are a handful of "healthcare" PR companies that work for drug giants such as Pfizer, GlaxoSmithKline, Merck and Astra Zeneca. The biggest, and most influential PR firms are Edelman, Ruder Finn and Chandler Chicco Agency in the United States and Medical Action Communications, Shire Health Group and Meditech Media in the U.K. One rule all these firms understand is that the best public relations go unnoticed. That way they are able to shape and mold our thoughts and attitudes without us even being aware of it. Perhaps the biggest illusion they perpetuate is that pharmaceuticals are remarkably safe and can miraculously restore health.

How do these firms create such illusions? CMD says the pharmaceutical companies know the most effective way to create credibility for a product or an image is by using an "independent, third-party" endorsement. Let's face it: while we might be skeptical if a drug company trumpets their own product, if an independent research institute with a very credible sounding name produces a scientific report that says a certain drug is fantastic, we're more apt to believe it.

To portray their clients and their clients' products in the best light, public relations firms cultivate and put forth to the public "key opinion leaders" such as doctors. They crank out press releases quoting "key opinion leaders" and other "experts," which can easily substitute for news. Patient groups are created to develop "disease awareness campaigns" or provide emotionally charged testimony in favor of speedy regulatory approval of new drugs.

The healthcare PR firms also organize events like medical conferences that provide a platform for well-trained "product champions" to announce promising results of drug research.

Such results can be reported by medical journalists—which are also hired by these PR firms—in unsuspecting medical journals.

Healthcare PR firms also undertake conventional lobbying strategies, such as opposing restrictions on "direct-to-consumer" advertising, which allows companies to market prescription and OTC drugs using the same techniques as toiletry items. They can also move very quickly and deftly to "squash" any negative news about their clients, as well as to promote damaging news about others. Could it be this is a strategy being deployed against the dietary supplement industry? It's not at all beyond the realm of possibility.

We've All Seen the Ads

Pharmaceutical companies spend loads of money getting their ads just right. I'm sure you've seen them. We're all familiar with the TV announcer's speedy, rat-a-tat delivery that causes us to not notice that their cure for excessive knuckle hair will probably make us sit on the toilet all day. Or the print across the bottom of the screen is so tiny you'd have to log time on the Hubble Space Telescope to read it.

Then there's my favorite—the unnamed remedy:

Announcer (with colorful, blissful scenes in the background): "Ask your doctor if the little (insert favorite color here) pill is right for you."

Patient to doctor: "Tell me, Dr. Jones. Is the little (favorite color) pill right for me?"

Dr. Jones: "I don't know, Mr. Smith. Are you having cramps when you menstruate?"

Of course, dietary supplements play their own games. We've all seen the ads:

"Lose 50 pounds in one day while pigging out with our miracle fat-burning formula!"

or
"Grow hair (lose hair) where you want (where you don't want)!"
or
"And you'll have more women (men) chasing after you than you ever thought imaginable!"

Of course, all these ads, featuring a post office box in a city you can't find on MapQuest, contain one itsy, bitsy caveat: "These statements have not been evaluated by the Food and Drug Administration. This product is not intended to diagnose, treat, cure, or prevent any disease." Still, when it comes to slick, pervasive and effective marketing, the dietary supplement industry doesn't hold a candle to the pharmaceutical industry.

Junk Science

True scientific research begins with no conclusions. Real scientists are seeking the truth because they do not yet know what the truth is. Another way you can often distinguish real science from the phony version is that real science points out flaws in its own research. Phony science pretends there are no flaws.

More often than you'd think, corporate-sponsored research (as is much of the research used in the pharmaceutical industry) begins with predetermined conclusions. It then becomes the scientist's job to prove that these conclusions are true because of the economic upside that proof will bring to the companies paying for that research. If the researcher finds the desired results can't be proven, the study will never see the light of day. Even the most honest, sincere and professional scientists—and they are in the vast majority—fall prey to this. The scientists have little control over what happens to the research—whether it's published, how the results are interpreted, etc.—because the companies are paying for the research.

This is one of the key complaints in *Trust Us, We're Experts,* authored by John Stauber and Sheldon Rampton of the Center for Media and Democracy (CMD). The CMD serves as a resource for journalists, public-minded citizens and anyone else who wants to verify the accuracy of information provided by public relations firms. The Center was founded in 1993 by Stauber, a public-interest activist.

Unlike many so-called "experts," the Center's agenda is quite overt—to expose the shenanigans of the public relations industry, which pays, influences and even invents a startling number of those experts.

Rampton and Stauber say there are two kinds of "experts" in question—the behind-the-scenes PR spin doctors and the "independent" experts paraded before the public, scientists who have been hand-selected, cultivated, and paid handsomely to promote the views of corporations involved in controversial actions.

Rampton and Stauber talk about the movers and shakers of the PR industry, from the "risk communicators" (whose job is to downplay all risks) and "outrage managers" (with their four strategies—deflect, defer, dismiss, or defeat) to those who specialize in "public policy intelligence," such as spying on the competition.

Stauber says the most disturbing aspect is not a particular example, but rather the fact that the news media regularly fails to investigate so-called "independent experts" associated with industry front groups. As I said at the beginning of this chapter, they all have friendly-sounding names like "Consumer Alert" and "The Advancement of Sound Science Coalition." However, they fail to reveal their corporate funding and their propaganda agenda, which is to smear legitimate health and community safety concerns as "junk-science fear-mongering" by criticizing, deflecting and making light of serious issues that raise questions about their clients.

Here's a great example of how this works. In a July 5, 2003 article of the *Atlanta Journal and Constitution* entitled,

"Chewin' the Fat: Whose Fault is Obesity?" the following quotes appeared. (Since this is simply an example, how you personally feel about the topic is less important than to note who is willing to comment.) Who do you think said the following?

"Pretty soon the only foods we'll be allowed to enjoy are locally grown organic bowls of steam."
"If we ban Coke, shouldn't we also ban orange juice from school vending machines?" and,
"If you eliminated fast-food stores I have sincere doubts that it would abate obesity."

The first quote was from Mike Burita, spokesman for the aforementioned Center for Consumer Freedom. The others come from Ruth Kava, director of nutrition at the infamous American Council on Science and Health. See how it works? Deflect, make light and criticize. And Stauber says the situation is only getting worse. More and more of what we see, hear and read as "news" is actually bogus PR content.

Strange Bedfellows

Corporate sponsors currently have formed "partnerships" with a number of leading nonprofit organizations, which allows them to pay for the right to use the organizations' names and logos in advertisements. Bristol-Myers Squibb, for example, paid $600,000 to the American Heart Association for the right to display the AHA's name and logo in ads for its cholesterol-lowering drug Pravachol. The American Cancer Society reeled in $1 million from SmithKline Beecham for the right to use its logo in ads for Beecham's NicoDerm CQ and Nicorette anti-smoking aids. A Johnson & Johnson subsidiary countered by shelling out $2.5 million for similar rights from the American Lung Association in its ads for Nicotrol, a rival nicotine patch.

The organization Consumer Alert frequently pops up in news stories about product safety issues. What the reporters almost never mention is that Consumer Alert is funded by corporations and that its positions are usually diametrically opposed to the positions taken by independent consumer groups such as Consumers Union.

In the early 1990s, tobacco companies secretly paid thirteen scientists a total of $156,000 to write a few letters to influential medical journals. One biostatistician received $10,000 for writing a single, eight-paragraph letter that was published in the *Journal of the American Medical Association.* A cancer researcher received $20,137 for writing four letters and an opinion piece to the British medical journal *Lancet,* the *Journal of the National Cancer Institute,* and the *Wall Street Journal.* And the scientists didn't even have to write the letters themselves. Two tobacco-industry law firms were available to do the actual drafting and editing.

When the Justice Department began antitrust investigations of the Microsoft Corporation in 1998, Microsoft's public relations firm countered with a plan to plant pro-Microsoft articles, letters to the editor and opinion pieces all across the nation, crafted by professional media handlers but meant to be perceived as off-the-cuff, heartfelt testimonials by "normal people."

These are examples of organizations relying on the public relations strategy known as the "third-party technique." Merrill Rose, executive vice president of the Porter/Novelli PR firm, explains the technique succinctly: "Put your words in someone else's mouth."

How effective is this strategy? According to a survey commissioned by Porter/Novelli, 89 percent of respondents consider "independent experts" a "very or somewhat believable source of information during a corporate crisis." Sometimes the technique is used to hype or exaggerate the benefits of a product. Other times it is used to create doubt about a product's hazards, or about criticisms that have been made of a company's business practices, all the while making it appear that the viewpoint is an "independent" one.

We used to see this technique in its most obvious and crude form in the television commercials that featured actors in physicians' lab coats announcing that "nine out of ten doctors prefer" their brand of aspirin. But advertisements are obvious propaganda, and the third-party technique in its more subtle forms is designed to prevent audiences from even realizing what they are experiencing.

"The best PR ends up looking like news," Stauber says a PR executive once boasted. "You never know when a PR agency is being effective; you'll just find your views slowly shifting."

Drug Media Bias

A study of how the mainstream mass media covers health topics discovered that many news stories on drugs fail to report side effects or state the researchers' financial ties to the companies that produce the medications. The authors of this study, whose findings appeared in a 2002 issue of the *New England Journal of Medicine,* analyzed 207 newspaper and television stories from 1994 to 1998 that dealt with three drugs: aspirin, Zocor, a cholesterol-lowering drug, and Fosamax, an osteoporosis drug.

In the 170 stories that cited experts or scientific studies, half included at least one expert or study with financial ties to the drug's manufacturer. Of those, only 40 percent reported the potential conflict of interest. The study also found that fewer than half the news stories reported the drugs' side effects and only 30 percent noted their cost.

Additionally, forty percent of the stories studied did not report the numbers behind the claims of medical benefits. Also, while 83 percent of the studies reported only the relative benefit, only 2 percent reported only the absolute benefit. A mere 15 percent reported both.

Why is this important? Reporting only the relative benefit is an approach that has been shown to increase the enthusiasm of doctors and patients for long-term preventive treatments and that could be viewed as potentially misleading. For example, many 1996 stories about a Fosamax study said the drug would cut an osteoporosis patient's risk of a broken hip in half—the relative benefit. But most failed to include the absolute reduction in risk, from a 2 percent chance of a hip fracture to 1 percent. Doesn't sound quite as good as the "cut in half" slant, does it?

(An interesting sidenote to this story is that the findings were published in the *New England Journal of Medicine,* whose incoming editor has been charged by the FDA for an apparent conflict of interest involving a drug company. He has admitted that he may have made a mistake last year when he praised a new asthma drug made by a company that had hired him to evaluate studies about the medication.)

How Drug Companies Create "Buzz"

In an article they contributed to the trade magazine PharmaVoice, Bob Chandler and Gianfranco Chicco explained that the key to promoting drugs is creating "buzz." They say while buzz should always appear to be spontaneous, it should, in fact, be scientifically crafted and controlled as tightly as advertising in the *New England Journal of Medicine.* Chandler and Gianfranco Chicco should know. In 1997 they teamed up to form the Chandler Chicco Agency (CCA), which now has offices in New York and London and is ranked among the top healthcare PR companies. CCA has plenty of experience creating "buzz," having launched Pfizer's $1 billion-a-year impotence drug, Viagra, and the wildly successful arthritis drug, Celebrex, for Pharmacia and Pfizer.

One of the reasons for Viagra's success, they explained, was

"Pfizer's sensitive and responsible approach" to encouraging potential patients to talk openly about impotence. To create "disease awareness," they hired celebrities and public officials to talk publicly about "erectile dysfunction," their preferred terminology.

"The buzz spread through the media, virtually eliminating the taboo word 'impotence,'" they wrote. In the U.S., they hired former Vice President Bob Dole to endorse the product, turning Viagra into a "success beyond a marketer's wildest dreams."

Pfizer's front group, Impotence Australia (IA), launched an advertising campaign with PR support from Hill & Knowlton. The campaign hit a snag, however, when its undisclosed ties to Pfizer were detailed in separate articles in *Australian Doctor* and the *Australian Financial Review.* Ray Moynihan, the author of the AFR story, revealed that Pfizer had bankrolled Impotence Australia to the tune of $200,000 Australian dollars (US $121,000). In an interview with Moynihan, IA Executive Officer Brett McCann admitted, "I could understand that people may have a feeling that this is a front for Pfizer."

A later Impotence Australia advertising campaign featured Pele, the Brazilian soccer legend. "Erection problems are a common medical condition but they can be successfully treated. So talk to your doctor today—I would," Pele advised.

When No News Is Good News

While some PR firms work to gain media profile for their clients, others endeavor to shut down bad publicity. In January 2003, for example, pharmaceutical companies were caught by surprise when the *British Medical Journal* featured an article by Moynihan challenging the use of exaggerated statistics by corporate-sponsored scientists seeking to create a new medical "syndrome" called "female sexual dysfunction."

Moynihan's article was picked up by hundreds of other publications around the world, prompting a hasty response by Michelle Lerner of the bio-technology and pharmaceutical PR company HCC DeFacto. Lerner, a former business reporter for *Miami Today,* scrambled to mobilize "third party" allies. She dispatched an email to a number of women's health groups.

"We think it's important to counter (Moynihan) and get another voice on the record," the email stated. "I was wondering whether you or someone from your organization may be willing to work with us to generate articles in Canada countering the point of view raised in the *BMJ.* This would involve speaking with select reporters about [female sexual dysfunction], its causes and treatments," she wrote.

Inadvertently, a copy of Lerner's email was forwarded to Moynihan. He contacted Lerner, who refused to disclose the identity of her client, stating that doing so would "violate ethical guidelines."

Writing for the *British Medical Journal,* Moynihan joined physicians David Henry and Iona Heath in warning that drug company marketing campaigns over-emphasize the benefits of medication. "Alternative approaches—emphasising the self-limiting or relatively benign natural history of a problem, or the importance of personal coping strategies—are played down or ignored," they wrote.

It is commonly believed that drugs are developed in response to disease. Often, however, the power of big pharma PR creates the reverse phenomenon, in which new diseases are defined by companies seeking to create a market to match their drug.

The healthcare PR practitioners are sometimes quite candid as they discuss the art of creating a need for a new product. "Once the need has been established and created, then the product can be introduced to satisfy that need/desire," states Harry Cook in the Practical Guide to Medical Education, published by the U.K.-based *Pharmaceutical Marketing* magazine.

Occasionally, patient groups are created to boost a new drug that is about to emerge from a drug company's "pipeline."

Most often, however, drug companies woo existing nonprofit patient groups. "Partnering with advocacy groups and thought leaders at major research institutions helps to defuse industry critics by delivering positive messages about the healthcare contributions of pharma companies," explains Teri Cox from Cox Communication Partners, New Jersey, in a September 2002 commentary in *Pharma Executive*. Corporate-sponsored "disease awareness campaigns" typically urge potential consumers to consult their doctor for advice on specific medications. This advice works in tandem with corporate efforts to influence doctors, the final gatekeepers for prescription drugs.

Julia Cook of Lowe Fusion Healthcare says potential "product champions" and "opinion leaders" in the medical fraternity are critical to influencing doctors' thinking. "The key is to evaluate their views and influence potential, to recruit them to specially designed relationship building activities and then provide them with a programme of appropriate communications platforms," Cook wrote in the *Practical Guide to Medical Education.*

Recruiting potential supporters to participate in an advisory committee, she says, allows time to develop a closer relationship and evaluation of how they can "best be used." However, a delicate touch is required. "Credibility can also be undermined by overuse," Cook warned. "If you front the same people to speak at your symposia, write publications, etc., they will inevitably be seen as being in your pocket."

Obtaining favorable coverage in medical journals is also an important element in pharmaceutical marketing. An investigation detailed in the *Journal of the American Medical Association* found that it was a common practice for articles to be "ghostwritten" for well-respected medical researchers.

In Oxford, England, 4D Communications is one of the PR firms that helps, in the words of its own website, to "mix experienced scientists with marketers and creatives to create memorable educational and commercial programmes." According to Emma

Sergeant, 4D's managing director, PR companies can help with the "creation of authoritative journals." Indeed, drug company-sponsored publications are so lucrative that in 1995 Edelman established a subsidiary company, BioScience Communications, to "meet the education needs of major pharmaceutical firms."

Journals, though, can achieve far more than touting the benefits of a new drug. Publications can be used to create a market "by creating dissatisfaction with existing products and creating the need for something new," wrote Harry Cook, of ICC Europe, in a medical publishing guide. "Reprints of journal articles can be a very powerful selling tool, as they are perceived as being independent and authoritative." This perception of independence and authority is precisely what healthcare PR firms use to keep the public from realizing that much of what they see, hear and read about drugs originates from sources beset with conflicts of interest.

In creating or co-opting patient groups, hiring "product champions" and cultivating doctors, PR companies make it difficult for consumers to obtain accurate, genuinely independent information that enables them to make informed health decisions. While healthcare PR campaigns are undoubtedly effective in selling more drugs, they don't necessarily make for a healthy population.

Then There's the Ephedra Industry

Ephedra has its own trade organization, which falls somewhere between the obvious ones such as the dairy industry and the not-so-obvious ones. While the Ephedra Education Council makes no bones about what product it represents, the "education" it provides about ephedra is purely one-sided: that ephedra is getting a bum rap.

Conversely, the EEC is candid about its mission and where its financial support comes from, listing all its members—all are

How to Spot the Phonies

Is it possible to tell which groups are on the up-and-up? Many do a good job of shielding themselves from scrutiny, but there are a few areas to look at that often yield warning signs:

· Who are its leaders and advisors?
· How is it funded?
· Does it oppose proven public health measures?
· Does it espouse a version of "freedom of choice" that would abolish government regulation of the health marketplace? Such "freedom" is nothing more than a ploy to persuade legislators to permit the marketing of questionable products without legal restraints.
· Is it a real organization? Sometimes names including "association" "institute," "clinic," or "laboratory" are nothing more than shady characters with a P.O. Box.
· Does it use outlandish claims in its marketing?
· Does it claim an affiliation, such as with a university you never heard of or a group whose name is *almost identical* to that of another credible organization?

dietary supplement manufacturers and distributors—on its site. While the EEC doesn't feature negative views about ephedra, it does provide references and links to actual studies in support of ephedra, rather than featuring PR spin.

Money Talks

The amount of money that EEC—in fact, all dietary supplement companies—spend to win friends and influence people pales in comparison to those that push pharmaceutical products. In fact, claims that ephedra manufacturers and marketers have paid for acceptance by getting politicians to look the other way, by contributing money to politicians, is laughable. As I said before, according to Federal Election Commission data compiled by the Center for Responsive Politics, the pharmaceuticals/health products industry contributed $26,941,139 to political campaigns in the 2002 election cycle. During the same period, nutritional and dietary supplement companies contributed $969,642—less than 4 percent of the amount contributed by the pharmaceutical industry.

The disparity is even more pronounced after subtracting political contributions by Metabolife, which appears on both lists (number 13 on the pharmaceutical list, number 1 on the dietary supplement listing—see the sidebars on the following pages). Metabolife, which has generated as much if not more heat and controversy due to its questionable behavior than any other ephedra company, contributed $847,750 to political campaigns. When their contributions are subtracted from both lists, Dietary Supplement political contributions are a paltry $121,892—less than one half of one percent of the pharmaceutical industry contributions.

By the way, if you look at the Pharmaceuticals/Health Products list in the following sidebar, you'll see at the very top—above familiar names such as Pfizer, Bristol-Myers Squibb, and Eli Lilly & Co—an organization with an innocent sounding name: the Pharmaceutical Research & Manufacturers of America. Better known as PhRMA, and representing a virtual "Who's Who" in drug companies, this organization gave more than $3 million in political campaign contributions in 2002, far and away the largest amount of any individual drug or dietary supplement company. In addition to individual drug company contributions, PhRMA wields a lot of political weight in various ways, from fighting DSHEA to making sure Medicare drug benefits don't allow American seniors' buying power to influence what the United States government pays for drugs, as is done in Canada and other countries.

Top Contributors of Political Donations within Pharmaceuticals/Health Products Industry, Election Cycle 2002

Total contributed: $26,941,139

Contributions from individuals: $3,072,303

Contributions from PACs: $6,939,382

Soft money contributions: $16,929,454

Rank	Organization	Amount	Dem	Repub
1	Pharmaceutical Rsrch & Mfrs of America	$3,180,552	5%	95%
2	Pfizer Inc	$1,804,522	20%	80%
3	Bristol-Myers Squibb	$1,590,813	16%	83%
4	Eli Lilly & Co	$1,581,531	25%	75%
5	Pharmacia Corp	$1,480,241	22%	78%
6	GlaxoSmithKline	$1,301,438	22%	78%
7	Wyeth	$1,188,919	17%	83%
8	Johnson & Johnson	$1,075,371	39%	61%
9	Schering-Plough Corp	$1,057,978	21%	79%
10	Aventis	$954,349	22%	78%
11	Amgen Inc	$913,242	24%	76%
12	Kinetic Concepts	$866,250	0%	100%

13	Metabolife	$847,750	60%	40%
14	Novartis Corp	$651,776	22%	78%
15	Abbott Laboratories	$648,967	7%	93%
16	Merck & Co	$622,817	23%	77%
17	Baxter International	$440,360	19%	80%
18	Genentech Inc	$285,515	43%	57%
19	Barr Laboratories	$276,401	22%	78%
20	Invitrogen Corp	$267,710	100%	0%

All donations took place during the 2001–2002 election cycle and were released by the Federal Election Commission on Monday, April 28, 2003. Feel free to distribute or cite this material, but please credit the Center for Responsive Politics.

Top Contributors of Political Donations within Nutritional & Dietary Supplement Industry, Election Cycle 2002

Total contributed: $969,642

Contributions from individuals: $187,775

Contributions from PACs: $20,367

Soft money contributions: $761,500

Rank	Organization	Amount	Dem	Repub
1	Metabolife	$847,750	60%	40%
2	National Nutritional Foods Assn	$19,367	62%	38%
3	Forever Living Products	$18,325	0%	100%
4	Yamanouchi Consumer	$13,750	85%	15%
5	SDA Enterprises	$12,000	83%	17%
6	Herbalife	$11,150	100%	0%
7	Longevity Science	$11,000	100%	0%
8	Great Lakes Capital	$9,500	21%	79%
9	D&F Industries	$8,000	100%	0%

The numbers on this page are based on contributions from PACs, soft money donors, and individuals giving $200 or more. (Only those groups giving $5,000 or more are listed here.) In many cases, the organizations themselves did not donate, rather the money came from the organization's PAC, its individual members or employees or owners, and those individuals' immediate families. Organization totals include subsidiaries and affiliates. All donations took place during the 2001-2002 election cycle and were released by the Federal Election Commission on Monday, April 28, 2003. Feel free to distribute or cite this material, but please credit the Center for Responsive Politics.

CHAPTER 7

Bad Medicine

IN MARCH 2000, Charles Young, of Pinole, California, began taking the prescription drug Baycol to reduce his cholesterol. Soon after he developed leg pains, which became so severe he could no longer walk. Not recognizing the cause of his patient's leg pains, Young's physician prescribed pain medication. Young's condition continued to deteriorate, and he was eventually admitted to the hospital. Within twenty-four hours he experienced complete kidney failure and was put on kidney dialysis. Not long after he suffered a severe heart attack and died on May 24, 2000.

What does Mr. Young's death have to do with ephedra? Nothing, technically. Rather it has to do with one of the arguments against DSHEA; particularly the intensive testing and approval process drug companies have to endure before they can get a new drug on the market. Since the rigorous testing is often held up as a model of how dietary supplements should be approved, monitored and controlled, let's take a look at how well the system is working.

Sadly, it turns out the death of Charles Young is one of multiple deaths and hundreds of serious injuries that have been reportedly linked to Baycol (cerivastatin). On August 8, 2001, the Food and Drug Administration (FDA) announced that Bayer Corporation, the manufacturer of Baycol, was removing the drug from the market because of reports of fatal rhabdomyolysis.

Rhabdomyolysis is a potentially life-threatening condition that occurs when a large number of skeletal muscle cells die, which results in the release of a massive amount of muscle protein (known as myogloblin) into the bloodstream. This muscle protein can become trapped in the kidneys, clogging up the filtering process of the kidneys and ultimately leading to their failure. In addition, potassium released from the damaged muscle cells can cause malignant heart rhythms, which results in cardiac arrest.

Soon after, the FDA received reports of thirty-two U.S. deaths due to severe rhabdomyolysis associated with use of Baycol, twelve of which involved concomitant gemfibrozil use. Outside the U.S., an additional twenty deaths associated with Baycol were reported. On January 18, 2002, Bayer announced that the estimated number of worldwide deaths linked to Baycol had risen to one hundred.

The Baycol recall lead to questions and governmental inquiries worldwide as to when Bayer was first aware that fatal side effects were associated with Baycol, and whether it failed to timely inform public health authorities of these side effects. (In the United States, the FDA does not provide any compensation to persons injured by recalled drugs.)

One of the principal allegations in the Baycol lawsuits is that following the drug's introduction, Bayer began receiving mounting clinical evidence and reports from physicians of serious side effects with the drug. At the same time, the plaintiffs allege that Bayer marketed Baycol as safe and highly effective while minimizing its risks, and that Baycol was no more effective than other anti-cholesterol drugs on the market. As a result, a number of lawsuits have been filed against Bayer for strict liability in its failure to warn, negligence and wrongful death.

Here's another example. In the July/August 1999 issue of the *Multinational Monitor,* of the top one hundred corporate fraudsters worldwide, Roche Pharmaceutical received the dubious distinction of being ranked #1 in the 1990s. Roche's frauds resulted in payments of approximately $10 billion to international suppliers and creditors it had defrauded. They also had to make payments of $500 million to the FBI, and paid fines of $462 million to EU authorities.

FBI and EU documents showed an extraordinary level of corruption, lies and misrepresentations made by Roche personnel at all levels of the organization, from its senior board of directors in Switzerland through the separate Roche board of directors in each of the countries where Roche conducted business. Roche senior directors and executives received personal fines and imprisonment. Their misdeeds were not only confined to financial misdealings but also to illegal medical fraudulent activities.

In one case Roche was found to have defrauded government health insurance programs by marketing a drug for medical conditions for which the drug had not received FDA license approval. A separate case involved payments by Roche subsidiary of $161 million in fines and penalties for participating in illegal "kick-back" payments to doctors. Other separate examples include illegal payments made by Roche and/or Roche subsidiaries to doctors in return for prescribing Roche drugs (under the guise that the doctors were conducting research, which research the authorities showed was not actually carried out by the doctors). A separate case involving payments by Roche of $11 million to the U.S. Heart Foundation who, after just one pre-trial study, endorsed the Roche product that was seeking a license for the treatment of heart disease.

A Congressional investigation found that Roche withheld safety information in its possession regarding another drug,

Versed, including reports of a number of Versed-associated deaths, as well as negative clinical trial data from the FDA. In the U.S., Roche also failed to pass on Adverse Reaction reports to the FDA.

In February 1998, the FDA applied increased label warnings for Accutane that featured psychosis and suicide as possible side effects. Roche immediately placed advertisements stating that acne causes depression, and that Accutane, by clearing acne, effectively relieved depression. The FDA was forced to issue two public letters to Roche about placing "false or misleading" material "to promote Accutane for an unapproved use in violation of the Federal Food, Drug and Cosmetic Act.

Corporate Welfare

For years, the pharmaceutical industry has benefited from a double standard of government protectionism and free enterprise; the federal government provides stringent intellectual property right protections and generous public subsidies for research—but does not regulate drug prices. As a result, the United States is on one hand a leader in the development of new drugs while on the other hand is faced with the highest drug prices in the world.

Until relatively recently, there has been little public controversy over the pricing of drugs or the terms under which private firms obtain the rights to government-funded research. But as health care costs have soared and policy makers attempt to deal with AIDS and the general crisis of health coverage and cost, the special treatment, power and control the drug companies wield shows that public interest and drug company interest collide more than intersect. And what's happening to counteract it? Virtually nothing.

An important part of this issue is how the government manages the transfer of publicly funded drug research and to what extent it regulates private companies that benefit from this transfer. The stakes are enormous. If we were to believe the drug companies, then government attempts to control drug prices would cripple the industry's research and development efforts, slow the pace of innovation, and damage one of the nation's leading high-technology export industries.

However, that really doesn't seem to be the case. Presently, the federal government funds about 42 percent of all U.S. health-care research and development (R&D) expenditures, including a significant portion of R&D costs for new drugs. The government plays a particularly important role in the highest risk research projects, including basic research, where commercial payoffs are least certain. It also pays a significant share of the later stages of drug development.

The Biggest Sham

Drug companies emphasize the high costs and risks associated with the development of new drugs and argue that these factors justify the policies concerning the transfer of government-funded technology to the private sector. However, while there is broad recognition that drug development is a risky and costly enterprise, there is considerable controversy over the methods used to "transfer" ownership of government-funded technology to the industry.

While the consumer advocacy group Public Citizen is no fan of DSHEA and ephedra, the organization—which was founded by Ralph Nader—goes ballistic when challenging the pharmaceutical industry.

For instance, a Public Citizen report released on Nov. 28, 2001 revealed how major U.S. drug companies and their lobby group, the Pharmaceutical Research and Manufacturers of America (PhRMA), have carried out a misleading campaign to scare policy makers and the public. PhRMA's central claim is that the industry needs extraordinary profits to fund expensive, risky and innovative research and development for new drugs. PhRMA's canned response goes something like this—If anything is done to moderate prices or profits, research and development will suffer, and, as PhRMA's president recently claimed, "It's going to harm millions of Americans who have life-threatening conditions." But this R&D scare tactic is patently untrue, says Public Citizen, and is built on myths, falsehoods and misunderstandings, all of which are made possible by the drug industry's staunch refusal to open its R&D records to congressional investigators or other independent auditors.

Using government studies, company filings with the U.S. Securities and Exchange Commission and documents obtained via the Freedom of Information Act, Public Citizen's report exposes as highly misleading the drug industry's claim that R&D costs total $500 million for each new drug (including failures). Extrapolated from an often-misunderstood 1991 study by economist Joseph DiMasi, the $500 million figure includes significant expenses that are tax deductible and unrealistic scenarios of risks. According to Public Citizen, the true figure is likely to be at least 75 percent lower—closer to $100 million.

Consider some of Pubic Citizen's other findings. Industry R&D risks and costs do not appear to be as risky as companies claim. According to *Fortune* magazine's rankings, the drug industry has been *the most profitable* in the United States every year since 1982. During that time, the drug industry's returns on revenue (profit as a percent of sales) have averaged about three times the average for all other industries represented in the Fortune 500. It defies logic that R&D investments are highly risky if the industry is consistently so profitable and returns on investments are so high.

Drug industry R&D is even less than they say, especially when considering that only about 22 percent of the new drugs brought to market in the last two decades were innovative drugs that represented important therapeutic gains over exist-

Who Is the Tufts Center for the Study of Drug Development?

The Tufts Center is primarily funded by large pharmaceutical companies, and it aggressively seeks corporate sponsorship, including for example several web pages that list the benefits of corporate sponsorship and glowing testimonials from big pharma CEOs. The Center routinely produces data that is used by big pharma companies in key Congressional debates over pricing and regulatory policies, and its study of drug development costs was announced by the CEO of Merck.

As the *New York Times* noted in a December 1, 2001 article entitled, "Research Cost for New Drugs Said to Soar," data for the study "were obtained from ten drug companies, and the Tufts center receives financial support from drug companies, among others."

ing drugs. Most were "me too" drugs, which replicated highly successful existing drugs.

In addition to receiving research subsidies, the drug industry is lightly taxed, thanks to tax credits. The drug industry's effective tax rate is about 40 percent less than the average of all other industries, according to the Congressional Research Service.

Sponsored by the pharmaceutical industry, in 1991 the Tufts University study pegged the average cost of developing a new drug at $231 million, based on industry data that reviewed the costs of clinical trials for ninety-nine new drugs. The Tufts study's $231-million figure has been widely misinterpreted. The study's authors found that the average inflation-adjusted cost of clinical research was about $20.4 million. The figure grew to $500 million by 2001, and PhRMA now boldly states today the cost of developing a new prescription drug exceeds $800 million.

But by including a number of adjustments, including the "dry hole" risks of failures and the opportunity costs of capital (foregone profits) the researchers came up with a figure of approximately $75 million. To get the $231 million figure, the Tufts researchers added $156 million, which they estimated to be the cost of pre-clinical research, adjusted for inflation, the cost of capital, and the risk of failure. The $156 million for pre-clinical research, however, was not supported by project level data, but was calculated on the basis of very rough aggregated data, with a mix of bold guesses.

While the industry has used the Tufts study to emphasize the high costs of drug development, it can also be used to argue that the prices for drugs developed with federal funds should be priced much lower than drugs developed without federal funding.

If, for example, the government has funded the preclinical research, then two-thirds of the cost of developing a new drug has already been paid. And if the drug company obtains the rights to the drug after the conclusion of phase II trials, more than 84 percent of the development costs have already been covered.

The Tufts study also dramatically illustrates the significance of the point at which a company acquires the technology. Government-funded medical R&D typically focuses on the early stages of a drug's development, when the risks are the highest.

For many drugs, the government has paid for most or all of the pre-clinical research, and it frequently funds the development of the drug all the way through FDA Phase II and Phase III trials. In these cases, which are many, the drug should not be priced as though the firm had borne all the risks and made all the investments. After all, citizens should not have to pay twice for the development of the drug, first as taxpayers and then as health care consumers.

Says Public Citizen, "taxpayer-funded research has helped launch the most medically important drugs in recent years and many of the best-selling drugs, including all of the top five sellers in one recent year surveyed (1995)." An internal National Institutes of Health (NIH) document, obtained by Public

Citizen through the Freedom of Information Act, shows how crucial taxpayer-funded research is to top-selling drugs. According to the NIH, tax-funded scientists conducted 55 percent of the research projects that led to the discovery and development of the top five selling drugs in 1995. I can find no proof that PhRMA has not challenged the NIH document.

Current federal policies for managing what drug companies do with government research still reflect the priorities of the 1980s, where a commitment to corporate interests often came at the public's expense. Throughout the 1980s, lawmakers enacted a series of "technology transfer" laws designed to provide incentives for commercial development and to prevent foreign interests from benefiting from U.S.-funded research and development. These laws made it increasingly easy for drug companies to obtain exclusive rights to federal research without being subject to pricing controls.

Not surprisingly, PhRMA tried to discredit the Public Citizen report. In their repudiation, PhRMA claimed that Lehman Brothers Healthcare Group—a division of an investment banking firm—estimated that R&D costs had skyrocketed to $675 million per new drug. PhRMA also said that the Boston Consulting Group (a firm that offers strategic management advice to business) put current average development costs between $590 million to $800 million for new drugs.

Public Citizen's scoffed at PhRMA's reply. They pointed out that it is unclear in the Lehman Brothers estimate what the methodology is, where the numbers came from, whether the opportunity cost of capital is included, and whether the figures are pre- or post-tax. (Note: The latter two methodological issues were used by Public Citizen to critique PhRMA's $500 million per new drug claim.)

Also, this work did not appear to have been peer-reviewed. Public Citizen said one reason it was able to deconstruct the DiMasi study is because it was published in an academic journal and its methodology was clear, as was the source of its data.

They also noted the Lehman estimate includes a huge figure ($230 million) for screening and finding new drug leads. There is no mention of the key contribution the National Institutes of Health (NIH) makes to this part of the process. It also assigns stratospheric costs to clinical research ($169 million for *each* of phases II and III; DiMasi, by comparison, put all clinical *and* approval costs at $75 million in 1987, or $114 million in year 2000 dollars). A recent report by the Congressional Research Service found that Phase I costs were $10 million, Phase II costs were $20 million, and Phase III costs were $45 million.

More important, this same Lehman Brothers document stresses that R&D should become more efficient and cheaper with new technologies. "Access to these technologies has led to a growing school of thought that the cost of discovering new biological targets and the cost of creating drug leads is falling." In addition, another Lehman Brothers document predicts that the R&D cost per new chemical entity (NCE) will drop by $150 million between 1996 and 2005.

"PhRMA can't have it both ways," scoffed Public Citizen. "It can't use the high Lehman Brothers estimate and at the same time ignore the fact that Lehman Brothers say R&D costs will decrease by 25 percent in the next several years."

How We, the Citizens, Pay Twice for Drugs

According to the Consumer Project on Technology—another consumer advocacy organization—of the twenty-one most important drugs introduced between 1965 and 1992, fifteen were developed using knowledge and techniques from federally funded research. Of these, NIH research led to the development of seven drugs used to treat patients with cancer, AIDS, hypertension, depression, herpes, and anemia.

To fully grasp how this combination of government protection and free enterprise works, let's look at the case of the cancer drug Taxol. In the late 1980s, Taxol held great promise as an effective treatment for breast, lung, and ovarian cancer. Taxol's only approved source is the bark of the Pacific yew, a rare and slowly maturing tree that is found mostly on federal lands. Taxol was discovered, manufactured, and tested in humans by NCI over a thirty-year period. Early studies on cancer patients were carried out under government grants at a number of universities. By 1991 the federal government had completed Phase II clinical trials on six types of cancer, and had plans to test Taxol on twenty-four more.

Rather than allow a group of companies to compete in developing Taxol, NCI decided to award the rights to a single firm in the form of a CRADA (Cooperative Research and Development Agreement; CRADAs are an agreement between federal agencies and firms outlining the terms of joint research efforts). The notice for the CRADA was published in the Federal Register in August 1989, and firms were given just 45 days to respond, despite the complexity of the CRADA proposal. Four companies responded.

The winning "bidder" was Bristol-Myers, a firm that was particularly well prepared, due largely to the fact that it had hired an NCI official, Dr. Robert Wittes, who had knowledge of the NCI Taxol program. The Bristol-Myers "bid" was submitted jointly with Hauser Chemical company, the firm that was then under contract to NCI to manufacture Taxol for the government's clinical trials.

The Bristol-Myers/NCI CRADA gave the firm exclusive rights to NCI's government-funded research, including the records of research completed before Bristol-Myers entered the Taxol picture, as well as all "new studies and raw data" from future NCI-funded Taxol research, which NCI agreed to make "available exclusively to Bristol-Myers," so long as the company is "engaged in the commercial development and marketing of Taxol."

According to Dr. Samuel Broder, Director of NCI, the federal agency was "totally responsible" for the development of Taxol, including the collection of the yew bark; all biological screening in both cell cultures and animal tumor systems; chemical purification, isolation, and identification; and sponsorship of all clinical trials. Broder has estimated the taxpayers will spend an additional $35 million on past and future Taxol research.

Just so you know, a full course of treatment with Taxol can cost between $10,000 and $20,000. Since its approval, Taxol has garnered an average of *$1 billion a year* to the Bristol Myers Squibb monopoly. In return, the government receives no money or royalties, but only Bristol-Myers Squibb's "best efforts" to commercialize Taxol, including a commitment to supply Taxol for government-run clinical trials, which were needed to obtain FDA marketing approval for the drug, and to an ambiguous "fair pricing" clause for Taxol.

If you think Taxol was a rare exception because of the urgency to develop the drug, think again. In 1998 the *Boston Globe* newspaper reported the National Institutes of Health (NIH) laboratories spent $1 billion on drug and vaccine development in the 1996 tax year, but only took in $27 million in royalties.

Convincing People to Buy

Marketing works, no question about it. According to a study in the *New England Journal of Medicine,* in 2000 drug companies spent $2.5 billion advertising their drugs to consumers. This year, they are expected to spend over $3 billion to convince you that their drugs are good for you. That does not even factor in the hidden subsidies to researchers that make the national news, which provides effective publicity—essentially "free advertising" for the drug companies.

Only the United States and New Zealand permit advertising of prescription medicines to consumers. The advertising has grown more controversial as both the number of ads and spending on prescription drugs continue to rise.

While $3 billion in advertising may seem like an awful lot, rest assured that the drug companies aren't worried. Why? Americans are expected to spend over $500 billion on drugs this year—not including the extra $100 billion estimated for the Medicare drug benefit program. Spending on prescription drugs is now the fastest growing portion of healthcare spending in the United States.

Some may argue that this increased advertising leads to increased awareness by consumers, and thereby improvements in their health. Unfortunately, this is simply not the case. According to the Harvard researcher who did the study, there is no solid evidence on the appropriateness of prescribing that results from consumers requesting an advertised drug.

Since the mid-1990s, pharmaceutical companies have tripled the amount of money they spend on direct-to-consumer advertising prescription drugs. From 1996 to 2000, totals rose from $791 million to nearly $2.5 billion. And despite the huge increase, drug companies spend even far more dollars in advertising their products to physicians, not consumers. The $2.5 billion figure for consumer ads is concentrated on a relatively small handful of medications.

Some physicians and health professionals are concerned that advertising drugs and medical tests directly to consumers interferes with the doctor-patient relationship and may raise medical costs by trumpeting expensive new medications. This increase is due no doubt in part to a rise in the number of effective medications, but there is widespread concern that part of the increase is due to advertising of drugs that don't necessarily provide better care.

Though broadcast advertising of prescription drugs has been legal for years, guidelines released by the FDA in 1997 clarified the rules for advertising directly to consumers. According to these guidelines, drug companies can fulfill their obligations for informing consumers about prescription drugs by referring in advertisements to four sources of additional information: their doctor, a toll-free number, a magazine or newspaper ad and a website.

According to a report prepared by the National Institute for Health Care Management, a nonprofit research foundation created by the Blue Cross Blue Shield health insurance plans, the fifty most-advertised prescription medicines contributed significantly last year to the increase in the nation's spending on drugs. The increases in the sales of the fifty drugs that were most heavily advertised to consumers accounted for almost half the $20.8 billion increase in drug spending last year, according to the study. The remainder of the spending increase came from 9,850 prescription medicines that companies did not advertise, or advertised very little. The study attributed the spending increase to a boost in the number of prescriptions for the fifty drugs, and not from a rise in their price.

Among the other reasons for increased spending, the study said, are an aging population, newer drugs that are more expensive than older medicines, and an increased use of drugs for chronic conditions like asthma or heart disease that involve taking medicines over long periods.

According to the study, Vioxx, an arthritis drug sold by Merck & Company, was the most-heavily advertised prescription drug and also accounted for more of last year's increased drug spending than any other single drug. Merck spent $160.8 million to promote Vioxx to consumers—more than PepsiCo spent to advertise Pepsi or Budweiser spent to advertise its beer, the study said. With the help of the advertising, Vioxx sales quadrupled to $1.5 billion last year from about $330 million in 1999.

Celebrex, another arthritis drug, which is locked in a marketing battle with Vioxx, was the seventh most widely promoted drug to consumers and was the fourth-largest contributor to drug sales growth last year. Other heavily advertised drugs contributing to the rise in drug sales are the cholesterol-lowering drugs Lipitor, Zocor and Pravachol; Paxil and Prozac for depression; Claritin, Allegra and Zyrtec for allergies; and Prilosec for ulcers.

Overall, consumer drug advertising rose 35 percent in 2000 (to $2.5 billion from $1.8 billion) in 1999, according to the study. Two of the biggest drug companies, Merck and Pfizer, increased their advertising much more than the industry average. Merck's total spending on consumer advertising increased 118 percent, while Pfizer's spending almost doubled.

And if that weren't enough, the British pharmaceutical company GlaxoSmithKline spent more on consumer advertising than any other company. It spent $417 million on advertising last year—an increase of 40 percent from the previous year.

According to Public Citizen's Health Research Group, while drug advertising more than tripled in dollar volume between 1996 and 2000, the number of warning letters and notices of violation issued by the FDA has dropped sharply in recent years. From mid-2000 through mid-2001, the FDA took 74 enforcement actions, less than half (47 percent) of the 158 enforcement actions taken between mid-1997 and mid-1998.

This translates to a likelihood that prescriptions are being given for drugs that are more dangerous and less effective than patients—or even doctors—realize. Until changes are made, both physicians and patients will be harmed by prescribing decisions based on all-too-frequently generalized and misleading information from advertisements.

Public Citizen cites several causes for this drop in warnings and notice violations:

- A shortage of FDA investigators to monitor ads
- A lack of regulations specifically written for direct-to-consumer drug advertising
- The limited enforcement power of the FDA
- The inability of the FDA to impose civil monetary penalties

Drug Deals Gone Bad

Here's just a small sample of approved drugs that have caused problems after approval, and how the drug companies reacted:

· *Accutane Capsules (isotretinoin), Hoffmann-La Roche Inc. (Roche Pharmaceuticals):* Although Roche warns that Accutane can cause serious birth defects, for eight years after the drug was introduced in 1982, nearly two thousand pregnant women had abortions and of 383 babies born, almost half had birth defects.

· *Baycol (cerivastatin), Bayer Pharmaceutical Division:* The FDA announced on August 8, 2001 that Bayer is voluntarily withdrawing Baycol from the U.S. market due to reports of sometimes fatal rhabdomyolysis, a severe reaction from this cholesterol-lowering (lipid-lowering) product.

· *Duract (bromfenac sodium capsules), Wyeth-Ayerst Laboratories (division of American Home Products):* This painkiller was pulled due to severe hepatic failure, which resulted in four deaths and eight liver transplants. All but one of those twelve cases involved patients using Duract for longer than ten days—the maximum recommended duration of treatment. The exception involved a patient with pre-existing significant liver disease.

Long before the withdrawal, the FDA had warned the manufacturer about proper labeling of the product. More specifically, the FDA's reviewer of Duract, Dr. John E. Hyde, had warned Wyeth-Ayerst of potential severe side effects after long-term use. Wyeth-Ayerst failed to recognize the problem in its early stages. (It's probably fair to say that if Wyeth-Ayerst had properly warned patients of severe side effect due to using the drug for more than ten days, they would have made less than the $89.7 million in sales generated by Duract).

· *Propulsid (cisapride), Janssen Pharmaceutica, (division of Johnson & Johnson):* Propulsid was prescribed for many adults suffering the symptoms of nighttime heartburn and for many infants suffering from colic. However, after the FDA received numerous reports linking the drug to dangerous side effects—including at least one hundred deaths—the manufacturer announced in March of 2000 that Propulsid would no longer be marketed in the United States.

· *Fen-Phen, Pondimin (fenfluramine), Redux (dexfenfluramine), phentermine, American Home Products:* Pondimin and Redux were two of the most widely prescribed diet drugs in the U.S. In 1996, sales of Pondimin and Redux totaled an estimated 20.6 million prescriptions. Pondimin and Redux were often sold in combination with phentermine, the "phen" in the Fen-Phen combination. It is estimated that over six million persons took fen-phen (also spelled phen-phen or phen-fen) prior to the drugs' recall in 1997. During the period from March to August 1997, the Mayo clinic in Rochester, Minnesota observed and reported an association between the use of fenfluramine and/or dexfenfluramine and valvular heart disease ("VHD"). On September 15, 1997, AHP and the FDA announced that there would be no further sales of Pondimin and Redux in the United States. Phentermine, which was sold under several brand names, was not recalled.

Since the withdrawal, epidemiological studies have established a causal relationship between fenfluramine and dexfenfluramine and VHD. Epidemiological studies have also established that fenfluramine and dexfenfluramine cause a fatal disease known as primary pulmonary hypertension ("PPH"). Over three hundred deaths were linked to the popular obesity drugs. In January 2002, American Home Products settled a $3.75 billion lawsuit.

· *Proventil and Theophylline, Schering-Plough:* Drugmaker Schering-Plough Corp. was fined by the FDA $500 million as part of a broad settlement aimed at resolving quality-control problems at four of its factories. The FDA said that the consent decree covers problems found in the manufacturing of 90 percent of the company's drug products since 1998, and involves 125 prescription and nonprescription drugs.

As part of the decree, the company agreed to suspend manufacturing of seventy-three products and to pay an additional $175 million if it falls behind in its efforts to improve manufacturing practices. The company said consumers should remain confident of its products, which are now under increased FDA oversight.

The problems detected at the four Schering-Plough plants, in New Jersey and Puerto Rico, involved "manufacturing, quality assurance, equipment, laboratories, and packaging and labeling," according to an FDA statement. An FDA official said the problems had to do with the overall manufacturing practices and quality control, and that the safety and effectiveness of individual drugs were not necessarily compromised.

The company recalled inhalers in 1999 and 2000, and Sidney Wolfe of Public Citizen said that Justice Department officials questioned him about the contents of the audit and the albuterol problems. "This company for years has grossly neglected the manufacturing of many of its products," Wolfe said. "They were told to clean up their act years ago, but they didn't do it."

A review of published medical studies shows additional cause for concern. In one, consumers believed that the FDA reviews drug ads before they are published or aired and that only the safest and most effective drugs may be advertised.

Considering all this, is there any question why spending for prescription drugs is the fastest-growing category of health care expenditures? No wonder two-thirds of all doctor visits now end with the patient receiving some sort of prescription.

Congress Is Not Helping

Over the years, shortcuts in the safety review process began to occur when Congress, lobbied by the drug industry, began pressuring the FDA to get drugs out on the market more quickly. Some members of Congress swallowed the big lie that most of these drugs were medical "breakthroughs."

That talk of breakthroughs is pure bunk. The vast majority of drugs that the FDA reviews and then approves are knockoffs of drugs already available to consumers. In any given year, only a few new drugs are truly in the "breakthrough" category.

To add insult to injury, the drug industry fought, and won, a nine-year legal battle to keep congressional investigators from the General Accounting Office from seeing the industry's complete R&D records. According to a report by the Congressional Office of Technology Assessment, Congress, which can subpoena the records, for some reason has failed to do so. Could it be because in 1999–2000 the drug industry spent $262 million on federal lobbying, campaign contributions and ads for candidates thinly disguised as "issue" ads?

Same Ol', Same Ol'

Naturally, the exposés by Public Citizen and others immediately changed everything, right? Wrong. Not when you're dealing with an organization with much deeper pockets for marketing, self-promotion and political contributions than its critics. Frankly, PhRMA has the resources to drown out any warning or plea Pubic Citizen and other consumer watchdog organizations try to make.

In July of 2003, PhRMA had this at the top of their website:

Most Drugs Never Recoup the Average Cost of Development:
The research-based pharmaceutical business is a long,
expensive and risky road . . .

In 2002, PhRMA member companies spent an estimated $32 billion on R&D, compared to the entire NIH operating budget of $24 billion. However, this investment does not fully reflect the chancy endeavor that makes our life-enhancing research such a difficult venture. PhRMA companies also invested more in R&D not only to improve the current rate of finding innovative medicines, but to meet the rising cost of bringing a drug to market. Economists recently published a new study finding that the average cost of developing a new prescription medicine was $802 million.

In addition, only three out of every ten drugs brought to market generate enough revenue to recover the average cost of its development. That means seven out of every ten drugs brought to market never generate enough revenue to recover the average cost of development.

There it is again—the $800 million figure out there for all the world to see. "It is impossible to say anything specific about the $802 million, because they have released nothing that explains the empirical basis for the number," said James Love, director of the Consumer Project on Technology. "It is a 'trust us' estimate at this stage. Later, once the number is burned into everyone's brain, we'll see the details.

CHAPTER 8

Drugged with Power

IT'S VIRTUALLY IMPOSSIBLE to walk around the nation's capital without tripping over a lobbyist representing some issue or industry. And, among them no industry wields as much power as the Pharmaceutical Research and Manufacturers Association (PhRMA), a pressure group known for its deep pockets and highly aggressive style.

Lobbying efforts by all industries in Washington, D.C., appeared to dip in the last couple of years due to the slumping U.S. economy. But the biggest drug companies showed no signs of cutting back on their lobbying. Instead, they increased their lobbying expenditures and number of lobbyists in 2001. PhRMA alone increased spending from $7.5 million in 2000 to $11.3 million in 2001—a 51 percent increase.

But when it came to lobbying for drugs, PhRMA wasn't alone. Consider these numbers:

• Companies that significantly hiked their lobbying expenditures in 2001 were GlaxoSmithKline (28 percent jump), Eli

Lilly (23 percent), Hoffman-LaRoche (23 percent), and Johnson & Johnson (17 percent).

- Four companies and PhRMA employed more than fifty different lobbyists in 2001. Pfizer and PhRMA employed the most (each hired eighty-two lobbyists), followed by Bristol-Myers Squibb (seventy-six lobbyists). Eli Lilly and Amgen each fielded fifty-eight lobbyists.
- The companies employed 623 different individual lobbyists in 2001—or more than one lobbyist for every member of Congress.
- Of these lobbyists, 54 percent have "revolving door" connections; in other words, they previously worked in Congress or another branch of the federal government, which often allows them easy access to their lawmakers and their staffs. Twenty-three of the 623 lobbyists are former members of Congress. Thirty-two of the lobbyists worked for the two House committees writing the Medicare prescription drug legislation.

And what about the dietary supplement industry? They can only dream of wielding such power. In 2001, brand-name drug companies easily outgunned the generic drug companies and supplement manufacturers. Brand-name pharmaceutical companies accounted for 97 percent of all pharmaceutical lobbying spending ($75.7 million out of a $78.1 million total). Brand-name companies also employed nine lobbyists for every one employed by generic companies. The supplement industry had even fewer.

Of course, much of the lobbying was devoted to a few key issues debated in government; primarily new rules for generic drugs and a prescription drug benefit. But there's no doubt they were more than happy to push another issue, albeit more secretly, on their agenda—drastic changes in the Dietary Supplement Health and Education Act, which would hopefully result in new legislation called the Dietary Supplement Safety Act of 2003. Congress could rule on this new proposal at any time (it could have happened before you even read this), once the other key legislation PhRMA favors is dealt with.

Don't feel bad if you haven't noticed. The real debate has arguably not been put before the American public with any clarity, because the extent to which the pharmaceutical industry in the U.S. has been able to set the policy-making agenda remains invisible to the average voter.

How entrenched are the drug lobbyist groups in our nation's lawmaking bodies? A July 2000 report, "Addicting Congress: Drug Companies Campaign Cash & Lobbying Expenses," by Public Citizen, describes the cozy working relationship between politicians and the drug industry. These relationships involve workings in strategy sessions, close collaboration to craft legislation favorable to the industry and attack consumer-oriented bills, and a revolving door status between Congress and the industry. Although primarily focused on the battle for a pro-drug industry bill for a prescription drug plan, the report makes some other intriguing points.

- The drug industry is spending vast sums on lobbying to hire well-connected former members of Congress and key staff to promote its financial interests before Congress. Overall, the drug industry spent $235.7 million from 1997 to 1999 to lobby officials in Congress and the executive branch. This amount does not include tens of millions more spent on television, radio and newspaper ads, direct mailings and telemarketing efforts.
- On the Medicare drug benefit and pricing issue alone, companies have hired 297 lobbyists—the equivalent of one lobbyist for every two members of Congress, an astonishing rate of coverage.

But Public Citizen isn't alone in its view of drug lobbying as a thorny issue. Many other organizations are concerned. One of these, Common Cause, recently issued its own report documenting how brand-name drug companies spent more than a quarter of a billion dollars to lobby the federal government, and how those lobbying efforts were backed up by more than $21.4 million in soft money contributions to national party committees and more than $16.6 million in political action committee (PAC) donations to federal candidates. The report also details how the industry has created and used deceptively named front groups like "Citizens for Better Medicare" (CBM) to put a pro-consumer sheen on their pro-industry agenda. And that agenda, says the report, has resulted in higher costs for consumers, less access to affordable drugs for the sick and elderly, and special tax breaks for what is considered to be one of the world's most profitable industries.

By the way, CBM was founded and is funded by PhRMA and the drug industry. When it registered itself for non-profit status, CBM declared itself as a PhRMA affiliate. CBM does not have a big staff or extensive premises because 98 percent of the money coming in from the industry is funneled straight out to a single advertising producer, Alex Castellanos.

Before being accused of objecting to the basic American principal of making money, Common Cause Education Fund President Scott Harshbarger added, "No one faults this industry for its quest for reasonable profitability. But this is an industry that has used its political power to sabotage all efforts to reduce the cost of prescription drugs for American families—hurting our pocketbooks and jeopardizing our health."

According to Common Cause, Congress has responded to the industry's generosity with an overdose of special favors, generous tax breaks, and other favorable legislation. These include:

• *Patent extensions:* Congress has helped brand-name companies hold onto the patents for some of their most profitable products, preventing consumers from taking advantage of less expensive generic versions. Twice, legislation passed by Congress has helped Schering-Plough hold on to its patent on the popular allergy drug, Claritin, extending the company's monopoly on the drug for nearly four more years. Nevertheless, Schering-Plough has continued in its fight to retain its Claritin patent beyond the current 2002 expiration date.

• *Sponging on government research:* The industry has successfully fought efforts to restore rules requiring reasonable pricing for drugs developed with the help of government funding from the National Institutes of Health (NIH). (See Chapter 7's discussion of Taxol.) An amendment that would have forced drug companies to charge "reasonable prices" for government-aided drugs passed overwhelmingly in the House of Representatives— but was killed in the Senate in 2000.

• *Tax breaks:* The Congressional Research Service found in 2000 that the pharmaceutical industry was the most lightly taxed of all major industries—thanks in large part to custom-built tax breaks offered by Congress over the years. These breaks include a tax credit for research and experimentation, which the industry has been able to extend ten times—including to companies that charge U.S. consumers much more than they charge foreign consumers. Even when Congress has phased out a measure that disproportionately aids the pharmaceutical industry—like a tax break for companies with operations in Puerto Rico—Congress has done so on the industry's terms.

Congress Says "Buy"

Let's face it: drug companies are good investments, and it should come as no surprise when political officials own or have owned stock in pharmaceutical companies. However, industry observers frown on this practice. "Holding shares of such companies ipso facto raises the appearance of a conflict of interest by members of Congress," says Peter Eisner, managing director of the Center for Public Integrity. "A member of Congress should be above suspicion of conflict of interest, and drug companies are a prime example of an industry in which members of Congress are courted and lobbied and make decisions that affect the value of the stock."

David King, an associate professor of public policy at Harvard University's Kennedy School of Government, said he is less bothered if members of Congress own stocks in drug companies when they have little influence over legislation affecting the industry. But, he said, "a member on the House Commerce Committee or the Senate Finance Committee would be skating on thin ice to hold a lot of drug stocks right now, because they are the ones who will be debating and deciding prescription drug benefits."

Research Roulette

The influence of drug companies sometimes goes deeper than politicians. In a recent issue of the *New England Journal of Medicine*, an editorial written by the former editor Marcia Angell, M.D., discussed the extent to which academic medicine has become intertwined with the pharmaceutical and biotechnology industries, as well as the benefits and risks of this state of affairs.

Dr. Angell reported that the ties between clinical researchers and industry include not only grant support but also a host of other financial arrangements. These include researchers who serve as consultants, join advisory boards, enter into patent and royalty agreements, promote drugs and devices at company-sponsored symposium, and accept expensive gifts and trips.

Although most medical schools have financial guidelines, the rules are generally relaxed and not very strict, and are likely to become even more so, she says. And it is not just individual researchers who are affected. Entire academic institutions are becoming increasingly beholden to industry.

One of the excuses offered for the close ties are that they are necessary to bring new drugs and devices from the laboratory to the marketplace in an expedient manner. However, Dr. Angell largely disputes this assertion. Although outright financial grants might, if properly done, have this effect, she cites the fact that much of the financial rewards and incentives are given to individuals rather than the institutions. Companies may hire a researcher as a paid consultant to obtain his goodwill, rather than to use his expertise.

A separate report in the same issue of the *NEJM* makes the case that there is now considerable evidence that researchers with financial ties are more likely to report favorable results than those without such ties. Although this does not mean that they are necessarily being "bought" or bribed, the financial ties, along with a close relationship with a company, can have at least subtle influences on an expert's judgement.

Another issue brought up by Dr. Angell is the problem of conflict of commitment, meaning that faculty who engage in extensive work for the industry may not have the time to devote to their students or to their school's educational efforts.

Whose Words Are These, Anyway?

In the past, medical publication articles were written by a study's principal investigator. More recently, a practice that one might call the nonwriting author-nonauthor writer syndrome has developed. Many interviews conducted for a report appearing in the July 15, 1998 issue of the *Journal of the American Medical Association* showed the prevalence of this syndrome in publications of drug-trial reports, editorials, and review articles. The syndrome has two features: a professional medical writer ("ghostwriter") employed by a drug company (the "contract research organization," or CRO), or a medical communications company, which is paid to write an article but is not named as an author; and a clinical investigator ("guest author"), who appears as an author but does not analyze the data or write the manuscript. Ghostwriters typically receive a packet of materials from which they write the article, and they may be instructed to insert a key paragraph favorable to the company's product.

The nonwriting author, who may be uninvolved in the research and have been requested to author the article to enhance its prestige, has final control over the manuscript. But many of these authors are busy and may not perform a thorough review. This guest-ghost syndrome is a growing phenomenon, particularly in the commercial sector, where community-physician investigators have little interest in authorship.

In one study, 19 percent of the articles surveyed had named authors who did not contribute sufficiently to the articles to meet the criteria for authorship of the International Committee of Medical Journal Editors. Eleven percent had ghostwriters who contributed to the work but were not named as authors. In justifying the nonwriting author-nonauthor writer syndrome, one industry executive explained that professional medical (ghost) writers are well trained, that investigators may be too busy to write, and that "nonwriting authors" are at fault if they do not carefully review ghostwritten manuscripts. An alternative view, articulated by Eric Campbell of the Institute for Health Policy at Massachusetts General Hospital and Harvard Medical School, holds that "a manuscript represents the accumulation of the intellectual and physical processes conducted under the aegis of a study and should be produced by the people who have actually been involved in the design, conduct, and supervision of the research." Tim Franson, Vice President for Clinical Research and Regulatory Affairs at Eli Lilly, believes that "any parties, be they industry staff, investigators, or others who contribute to the content of articles, should have their names listed on the article."

No doubt that without industry funding, some important

advances in disease prevention and treatment would not occur. In the words of Lee Goldman, chairman of the Department of Medicine, University of California at San Francisco, "companies translate biologic advances into usable products for patients. They do it for a profit motive, but they do it, and it needs to be done." Investigators interviewed for this report confirmed that many collaborations with pharmaceutical companies were conducted on a highly professional level.

But when results are disappointing for a company, conflicts may develop. Dr. Curt Furberg, with years of experience in industry-funded drug trials, stated: "Companies can play hardball, and many investigators can't play hardball back. You send the paper to the company for comments, and that's the danger. Can you handle the changes the company wants? Will you give in a little, a little more, then capitulate? It's tricky for those who need money for more studies."

Although academic-industry drug trials have been tainted by the profit incentive, they do contain the potential for balance between the commercial interests of industry and the scientific goals of investigators. In contrast, trials conducted in the commercial sector are heavily tipped toward industry interests, since for-profit CROs and site management organizations (SMOs), contracting with industry in a competitive market, will fail if they offend their funding sources. The pharmaceutical industry must appreciate the risks inherent in its partnership with the commercial drug-trial sector: potential public and physician skepticism about the results of clinical drug trials and a devaluation of the insights provided through close relationships with academic scientists.

A number of authors have recommended changes to resolve the problems of clinical drug trials. An essential ingredient of any solution is increasing the independence of investigators to conduct and publish their research. Many industry observers believe that drug trials should be funded by industry, but they also feel that the design, implementation, data analysis and publication of such research should be controlled entirely by academic medical centers and investigators. The rise of the commercial sector—which reduces rather than enhances the independence of investigators—appears to be moving drug trials in the opposite direction.

Study Funding Should Be Made Public

Because private funding of medical research may lead to conflicts of interest in reporting findings, scientific journals should publish funding information along with their findings. And financial disclosures, where researchers state any potential personal gain from study findings, should also be published. Some authors point out that a recent survey reveals that just 26 percent of American medical journal editors specifically require that researchers submit information on funding as a condition to publication. And an even smaller percentage of editors required that authors supply information regarding their personal affiliation (employment by or stock ownership in, for example) with potentially influential institutions.

The bottom line? The financial underpinnings of medical research deserve very close scrutiny, especially now that competition for public and private research dollars has become so fierce. Pharmaceutical executives believe this competition has bred "a more entrepreneurial spirit" among scientists, as well as closer ties between academics and private industry. All I have to say is "money talks." Ignoring conflicts of interest in scientific research is a sticky ball of wax because the stakes in the drug business are a lot higher than in most other industries. Remember, the products this industry produces kill a lot of people each year. And quite often, the government officials who are entrusted with our safety from the pharmaceutical industry's greed often have their own pockets stuffed full of pharmaceutical money.

CHAPTER 9

Hearings or Witch-Hunt?

"THIS WEEK THE gentleman from Michigan (Mr. Dingell) and I and all of the members of the Committee on Energy and Commerce had to face a horrible realization: This week we faced the parents of Steve Bechler, the 23-year-old pitcher for the Baltimore Orioles, who died of a heart attack at that young age taking ephedra tablets, tablets which we in 1994 voted to exempt from FDA safety regulations. I have got that on my conscience now. In 1994, you and I decided, those of you who were here with me, that safety did not matter when it came to ephedra.

"Mr. Speaker, as the Justice Department criminal investigations are under way and as our own Committee's investigation is under way, we learned this week that over 17,000 serious events have occurred as a result of the use of unregulated ephedra; young athletes, young people, dying, suffering strokes, heart attacks, like Steve Bechler, because we voted in 1994 to say that safety did not count when it came to ephedra."

– *Billy Tauzin, U.S. Representative (R-LA), Chairman of the House Energy & Commerce Committee, July 25, 2003*

In July 2003, the U.S. House Subcommittee on Oversight and Investigations held two days of hearings. The official title of these hearings was "Issues Relating to Ephedra-containing Dietary Supplements." This Subcommittee falls under the auspices of the House Energy & Commerce Committee, which is led by Chairman Billy Tauzin.

The July 2003 hearings were vastly different in tone and substance from the August 2000 gathering at the FDA and CFSAN-sponsored meeting at the Office of Women's Health (OWH). That summer, a group of scientists, government officials, industry experts and interested parties met in Washington for two days of hearings about the safety and risks of ephedrine alkaloids. This time, not one member of the panel put together by the Ephedra Education Council were invited, nor were any of the other doctors who spoke in support of ephedra. Were they discredited in the ensuing three years, making their testimony suspect? Outside of receiving honorariums from the Ephedra Education Council—a fact none of them tried to hide—their testimony and research is still being cited. You may be saying to yourself, "But they were paid by a pro-ephedra organization—can we really trust their statements?" That's exactly the kind of question a House Subcommittee member might ask. But as you'll see later, the last people who should criticize the receiving of funds are many of the House Subcommittee members.

Let the Hunt—Uh, Hearings—Begin

The mood of the hearings was established before they even began. As a July 23, 2003 article in the *New York Times* stated while quoting "unnamed officials," "For several years, the industry had refused to give the regulators all the data from the study, which was conducted at medical centers in New York and Boston in the late 1990s. But last February, the Food and Drug Administration made an unusual deal to gain access to the data, officials say." The study the *New York Times* is referring to is the Boozer/Daly study.

The article, entitled "Expert Panel Finds Flaws in Diet Pill Safety Study" and written by Christopher Drew and Ford Fessenden, continues, "The agency had to make the deal, the officials say, because it was in a bind. While drug companies are required to prove the safety of their products and must turn over safety data and consumer complaints to the FDA, the agency, under a 1994 law, has no such authority over the makers of dietary supplements like ephedra.

"The notion that a federal regulatory agency had to make a deal to investigate a health threat also goes a long way, critics say, to explaining how the ephedra companies have been able to keep the government at bay through nearly a decade of complaints about their products."

At first, it appears the *New York Times* raises some interesting points, that is until you hear, as Paul Harvey likes to say, "the rest of the story." According to Dr. Boozer in a phone interview and emails we exchanged in early September 2003, she had told Metabolife before she conducted the first study that she planned to publish the results in a medical journal, regardless of the outcome. When she and an industry attorney struck a deal after many months of negotiation with the FDA for her data, the agreement was that the FDA would ask independent scientists to review the data. On top of this, the FDA agreed to provide her with copies of these reviews prior to the government making them public in any form. You can imagine her surprise when portions of their reviews showed up in the *Times* article before she saw them.

In the same *New York Times* article, the reporters also wrote, "Top agency officials said they agreed to the deal to counter industry concerns that the agency's scientists were biased against ephedra. Representative James C. Greenwood, a Republican from Pennsylvania and the chairman of the House subcommittee that will hold a hearing on ephedra today, said the deal made sense because the outside experts ended up show-ing that the study was 'seriously flawed.'"

Naturally Boozer was stunned when she read this, and two months later, still cannot get the *New York Times* to correct their article. Should they? I think they should, and not just based on what Dr. Boozer says. I saw the documents provided by the FDA to the House subcommittee.

Included with the reviews is a letter stamped May 14, 2003 from Charles W. Prettyman of HHS to FDA Commissioner Dr. Mark McClellan. There are two interesting points in this letter. First, as we already mentioned, the FDA had agreed to share the results of the reviews with Dr. Boozer and an industry lawyer *before releasing it to the public.* Yet, somehow the *New York Times* obtained them first. (In fact, when Dr. Boozer testified at the July hearings she *still* hadn't seen the reviews. The Prettyman letter was not made public until August 8.)

Second, in his letter Mr. Prettyman wrote:

> The main points I gather from the three reviews [one still hadn't come in] are as follows:
>
> • The study was generally well designed and conducted.
> • The formulation may or may not represent what is being marketed.
> • The controls, subject selection, exclusion criteria, and moni-toring do not represent real world use conditions.
> • The product seems to offer some short-term weight loss.
> • The product should only be used with the monitoring of a learned intermediary.
> • One expert believes the study was seriously compromised due to some mix-up in the active and placebo preparations.

Can't the *New York Times* distinguish between "expert" and "experts"? It makes a big difference. More later in the chapter. As I considered the concerns raised by the article and began reviewing the list of those scheduled to speak, I wondered why Dr. Wanda Jones, Deputy Assistant Secretary for Women's Health at NIH who headed the 2000 meeting, was not asked to testify at the current hearings. She certainly would be objective, I thought. But she wasn't invited. The truth is, when I further scrutinized the names of the presenters, I had a gut feeling this had the potential to be more a witch-hunt than objective inquiry.

Here's how James Greenwood, Chairman of the Subcommittee on Oversight and Investigations opened the meeting: "Good morning and welcome to the first day of hearings on issues relating to ephedra-containing dietary supplements. Baltimore Orioles pitcher Steve Bechler and high school athlete Sean Riggins probably thought they were helping themselves when they used ephedra supplements either to lose weight or enhance athletic performance. Tragically, these two young men, twenty-three years and sixteen years of age respectively, died. And coroners who investigated their cases believed ephedra played a role in their deaths . . ."

Could Mr. Greenwood have been any more blatant in his bias against ephedra? As they say, the die was cast.

I think it would be helpful to maintain a scorecard based on preconceived positions shared by those presenting, unless testimony proved otherwise. So, to begin (and we won't count Mr. Greenwood's opening):

Anti-Ephedra	0
Defended Ephedra	0

The first two witnesses were Pat and Ernie Bechler, parents of Steve Bechler. They were accompanied by their lawyer, Todd Macaluso. In June, the Bechler's filed a civil action charging wrongful death, product liability, negligence, fraud and misrepresentation against Cytodyne Technologies, Inc., and Phoenix Laboratories, the manufacturers of Xenadrine RFA-1, the diet supplement their son had been taking at the time of his death. Why did they need a lawyer there? Most likely to guide them in their responses in case questions were raised about a story appearing in the Sun-Sentinel of Fort Lauderdale in March. In the story, Mrs. Bechler said her son suffered "a couple of heat-strokes" while in high school. "He was probably sixteen, seventeen years old," Pat Bechler told the newspaper. "Both of them happened when he was playing baseball."

In an ESPN story run the same time, which also used Associated Press material, Ernie Bechler said Steve Bechler's half-brother, Ernie Jr., died at age twenty from a brain aneurysm. "He came in from playing baseball one day. He was hot, and he suddenly had a severe headache. He collapsed on the floor, and he was dead by the time the paramedics got there."

The Bechler's testimony was heart wrenching, with Mrs. Bechler tearfully asking how many others "will have to die to prove these products are not safe?" The Bechler's appearance set the tone for the entire hearing.

Anti-Ephedra	2
Defended Ephedra	0

The next witness was Mr. Kevin Riggins, father of the late Sean Riggins and Founder and Director of the Sean Riggins Foundation for Substance-Free Schools in Lincoln, Illinois. Here's part of what Mr. Riggins said:

"My wife and I were not familiar with this particular substance; in fact, we had no idea that Sean had been taking it. As we were to discover later through investigation and conversations with Sean's teammates, numerous teenagers, including athletes and young people trying to lose weight, were using these products. The teens could buy these pills at the corner gas stations with pocket change," he stated. "The little packages, which promote weight loss, performance and energy enhancement, were being sold right next to the Twinkies and candy bars. In fact, the use of these products was so casual, none of the kids believed that they were taking a drug. With the marketing style and the ease in which they could be obtained, the teens thought nothing of it. 'They sell these things in the stores, they are not illegal, so they must be okay.' This was a quote from one of my son's friends. As it turns out, the vast majority of the American public believes this as well."

Mr. Riggins then went on to bash DSHEA. Does any of this ring a bell?

> As Americans, we believe that our regulatory organizations, in this case the FDA, are protecting our interests by not allowing dangerous products to be sold, especially in regards to what we put in our bodies. In the case of ephedra, we could not be more wrong. As you well know, the Dietary Supplement Health and Education Act of 1994 allows dietary supplement companies to operate with virtually no federal oversight. A company does not need a license to produce these products, nor are there any no pre-market approval requirements. There have never been any Good Manufacturing Practice guidelines developed for these companies and they have a voluntary adverse event reporting system. When a supplement poses a risk of serious injury or death, the burden of proof falls to the Government to prove cause and effect. This is the exact opposite of the rules and regulations set up for drug companies.

Anti-Ephedra	3
Defended Ephedra	0

Mr. Riggins was followed by Mr. Michael Vasquez—along with his lawyer, Fred G. Cohen via satellite. In a court deposition the previous August, Vasquez, a nurse and former Metabolife employee, said the company had nurses on ten telephones receiving calls from consumers. He testified he handled about five adverse event calls per day. In an article appearing in the August 25, 2002 edition of the *Union-Tribune* of San Diego, Vasquez said one out of five calls were about cardiovascular symptoms, and during the four months he worked at Metabolife, he said he received about ten calls from emergency room physicians seeking information about Metabolife ingredients as they tried to provide emergency treatment to patients who had taken the pills and complained of illness.

Vasquez said all calls of serious consumer injury were forwarded to a Metabolife supervisor, and the reports were discussed with Metabolife's legal department at least once a week. In some cases, Metabolife footed the costs for emergency room treatments of some of its customers.

Anti-Ephedra	4
Defended Ephedra	0

Next up was Steven Heymsfield, M.D., Deputy Director of Obesity Research Center at St. Luke's-Roosevelt Hospital, where Dr. Carol Boozer worked. Here's part of his testimony:

"There exist three categories of chemical agents available for weight loss treatment. The first two categories are prescription drugs and over-the-counter drugs. The Food and Drug Administration (FDA) regulates these agents under carefully controlled guidelines for safety and efficacy. The process is particularly rigorous for weight loss agents.

"Prescription and over-the-counter drugs are rigorously tested, using modern scientific guidelines and procedures to ensure public and individual safety. In 1994 a third category of agents emerged referred to as "dietary supplements."

Dr. Heymsfield then talked specifically about ephedra:

I would now like to focus some specific comments on dietary supplements that include ma huang as the main active ingredient. I select ma huang because consumers are exposed with these products to a potentially dangerous family of ingredients, the ephedra alkaloids, that not only produce weight loss but that may lead to strokes and heart attacks with associated disability and death in selected susceptible patients.

A key concern is that overweight and obese patients are particularly vulnerable to taking purported dietary supplement weight-loss products because they are often desperate, want to lose weight quickly, find physician evaluations time consuming and costly, and have often tried dietary and medical therapies of limited current effectiveness.

By avoiding medical oversight, overweight and obese consumers purchasing dietary supplements make the false assumption that dietary supplements and herbal preparations are inordinately safe and may pose no or very little risk . . .

Later he said, "Given the well-recognized risks of this group of dietary supplements and the appropriate lack of interest in the area by pharmaceutical companies, there exist very few careful safety and efficacy trials that meet the current standards set forth for evaluation of pharmaceutical weight-loss agents.

"A concern regarding the well-controlled clinical trials is that subjects were appropriately medically screened prior to entry into the trial so as to reduce the medical risks of those exposed. One such trial was carried out at our institution and only those subjects deemed medically acceptable were entered into treatment."

While Dr. Heymsfield makes some valid points, it's important to note he is speaking prior to testimony scheduled later by his colleague, Dr. Carol Boozer. Dr. Boozer's clinical studies, which I reported on in Chapter 4, found ephedra to be safe. Dr. Heymsfield's testimony seems to downplay, if not refute, what she is prepared to say before she even gets to say it.

| Anti-Ephedra | 5 |
| Defended Ephedra | 0 |

Dr. Raymond Woosley, M.D., Ph.D., Vice President for

Health Sciences at the Arizona Health Sciences Center, University of Arizona, was next to speak: "I have consistently recommended that the FDA take steps to have non-prescription products containing ephedrine removed from the market. In 2001, I joined Public Citizen, a consumer advocacy organization, and filed a citizen's petition calling for an FDA ban on ephredrine-containing dietary supplements."

Enough said.

Anti-Ephedra	6
Defended Ephedra	0

Next was Douglas Zipes, M.D., Director of Division of Cardiology at the Krannert Institute of Cardiology, Indiana University School of Medicine in Indianapolis. "Laboratory analysis of these products has disclosed that there is considerable variation in the composition of herbal supplements from one manufacturer to another and often from lot to lot from the same manufacturer," he testified. "Most of these herbal products have not been tested rigorously, with the accepted norm of standardized, controlled, prospective, randomized trials that we use to test medical drugs and devices. In addition to lack of efficacy for the claimed use, some of these products produce important side effects either directly or by interactions between the herbal remedies and prescription drugs and over-the-counter (OTC) drugs."

Anti-Ephedra	7
Defended Ephedra	0

Dr. Cynthia Culmo, R.Ph., a former official with the Texas Department of Health followed. She discussed how the previous year, the Texas department, spurred by reports of more than seven hundred cases of side effects and eight deaths linked to ephedra, tried on several occasions to impose regulations that would have required a prescription to purchase ephedra products. At the time, there were charges the ephedra supplement industry mounted an intense lobbying effort, and Metabolife contributed generously to local politicians and helped bankroll lobbying efforts.

Anti-Ephedra	8
Defended Ephedra	0

Next to testify was Dr. Marcia Crosse, Ph.D., Acting Director of Health Care-Public Health and Science Issues in the U.S. General Accounting Office (GAO). "In summary, FDA has determined that dietary supplements containing ephedra pose a significant public health hazard based on the 2,277 adverse events reports it has received. The number of adverse event reports FDA has received for dietary supplements containing ephedra is fifteen times greater than the number it has received for the next most commonly reported herbal dietary supplement," she said. "While it is difficult to establish with certainty that a particular adverse event has been caused by the use of ephedra, based on the pattern of adverse event reports it has received and the scientific literature it has reviewed, FDA has concluded that ephedra poses a risk of cardiovascular and nervous system effects among consumers who are young to middle-aged." She then reported a total of five deaths attributed to ephedra.

I've already discussed the GAO report in Chapter 4, but one thing bears repeating—the GAO had found the AERs were insufficient evidence for the FDA to impose stricter limits on the amount of daily doses of ephedra.

Dr. Crosse also mentioned ephedra caused fifteen times more adverse effects than the next most common dietary supplement. This brings us to a study appearing in the March 18, 2003 issue of *Annals of Internal Medicine* entitled, "The Relative Safety of Ephedra Compared with Other Herbal Products." Commonly referred to as the "Bent Study," since the lead author's name is Stephen Bent, M.D., the study found the risk for adverse events attributable to ephedra accounted for 64 percent of all adverse reactions to herbal products in the United States, yet these products represented only 0.82 percent of herbal product sales. The researchers concluded "ephedra use is associated with a greatly increased risk for adverse reactions compared with other herbs, and its use should be restricted."

Not everyone concurs. Comments filed independently with the FDA set forth a rigorous critique of this article. Poison experts, including Richard Kingston, Pharm.D., Vice President and Sr. Clinical Toxicologist at PROSAR International Poison Center, and Associate Professor at the University of Minnesota, wrote that the authors of this paper committed serious errors, misrepresenting the data as well as committing methodological flaws. Regarding factual misrepresentations, these authors reported that "all the incidents that were tabulated under the ephedra containing product categories represented 'adjudicated' reports of adverse effects." The poison experts added, "They [the authors of the 'Bent Study'] failed to acknowledge that the vast majority of these calls undergo no process of authentication. As any poison center specialist who has ever fielded an exposure-related inquiry in a public poison center can attest, just mere fact that someone calls the poison center does not always mean that the event in question is accurately depicted or reported. In fact, these incidents are rarely verified by independent medical practitioners. More often than not, these incidents represent reports from the general public, often made anonymously, and typically accepted at face value."

Still, score one for the "home team."

Anti-Ephedra	9
Defended Ephedra	0

This ended the first panel. So far, the "Anti-Ephedra" team

had completely dominated the contest. In fact, the "Defended Ephedra" team hadn't even touched the ball.

Panel Two: Perp Walk

Any hopes of turning the tide in defense of ephedra with the second panel were dashed before the first word—or lack thereof—were uttered. Of the many companies selling ephedra products, the Subcommittee issued subpoenas for executives from only three:

- *Five officials from Metabolife:* More than eighty-five consumer lawsuits are now pending against the company.
- *One official from Cytodyne Technologies:* Manufactured the product implicated in the death of Steve Bechler.
- *Two officials from NVE Pharmaceuticals:* Manufactured the product linked to the death of Sean Riggins.

Before the hearing, FDA and HHS officials told the *New York Times* they were trying to determine whether Metabolife's founder, Michael Ellis, lied when he told the Food and Drug Administration in 1998 that the company had never received notice of "any serious adverse health event" among users of Metabolife 356, its flagship product, which contains ephedra.

As expected, Mr. Ellis, along with a former Metabolife chief executive, David Brown, and the company's head nurse, Daniel Rodriguez, all refused to testify at the hearing, invoking their Fifth Amendment right to avoid compelled self-incrimination.

K. Lee Blalack II, a lawyer for Mr. Rodriguez, said his client declined to testify because he was cooperating with Justice Department investigators. Mr. Blalack said Mr. Rodriguez has received immunity from prosecution.

Robert Occhifinto, the president of NVE Pharmaceuticals, acknowledged that he had twice been convicted of federal crimes, including selling raw materials to a maker of illegal drugs, and that his company had never employed a doctor or chemist in creating the ingredient formulas for its products.

Anti-Ephedra	17
Defended Ephedra	0

Dr. Carol Boozer was also a member of this panel, but they tried to sink her before she began. For one thing, they included her on the same panel as the ephedra-selling executives (whose problems we just documented). Was this a deliberate attempt at guilt by association?

Press reports prior to the hearing showed that experts hired by the FDA had found shortcomings in a study led by Dr. Boozer, saying supplement industry officials had promoted the study as suggesting that ephedra diet pills are safe.

Also prior to the hearings, the *New York Times* reported, "Documents released by Mr. Greenwood's subcommittee show that the three scientists hired to review the data all ended up criticizing the study. One of the agency's experts noted that through a mix-up, some of the participants who were supposed to receive placebos were given a mixture of ephedra and caffeine similar to what is in most of the diet pills, thus making the study 'impossible to rely on.'"

Let's go back to the letter from Mr. Prettyman of HHS, which stated, "The study was generally well designed and conducted." Adds Dr. Boozer, "The primary shortcomings cited were that the study would have been better if it were larger and longer—statements that are true about any study."

And what of the pill mixup? The article quotes one reviewer as saying that the amount of mix-up between the placebo pills and ephedra pills—which was only 1.5 percent of the total—made the study impossible to rely on. "But none of the other three reviewers (including one from the FDA) mentioned this as a problem," says Dr. Boozer. "The *New York Times* article also implies that it was the reviewer who found the problem, when actually, I was the one who found the error, investigated it and reported it to both the journal editors and the FDA—prior to initiation of the reviews." Dr. Boozer also indicated this was pointed out by one of the reviewers, Dr. Richard Atkinson, and by a colleague, Dr. Allan Geliebter, in a letter to the Editor of the *Times,* published on July 26.

The *Times* article continued, "Another FDA expert, Dr. Norman Kaplan, a hypertension specialist at the University of Texas Southwestern Medical Center at Dallas, said that with only 87 participants completing the six-month study, the group was too small to assess safety. He also said the researchers had played down increases in heart rates and blood pressure among study participants, which could translate into a 20–40 percent increase in strokes and heart attacks among ephedra users."

Dr. Boozer points out the article failed to mention that another reviewer, Dr. Atkinson, stated that these changes were "clinically insignificant." "The truth is that scientists differ in their interpretation of the clinical relevance of these changes," says Dr. Boozer.

Again, the *Times:* "In addition, the reviewers said the study would be a poor predictor of what might happen to the general public. Two reviewers noted that the study enrolled only people in near-perfect health, using a series of rigorous tests to eliminate 11 percent of the volunteers before the trial began."

To this point, Dr. Boozer responded, "It is standard practice in clinical trials to screen out individuals who are not healthy to avoid exposing such individuals to potential risks, and to avoid confounding the results."

Although she defended her studies during her testimony, Dr. Boozer concluded with the following statement:

> While efficacy of ephedra in promoting weight loss is established, it is not my position that the safety of herbal ephedra is proven for different populations or with different usage.

Additional research would be required to determine effects in people who are not healthy, or who consume ephedra at levels above those studied, or for periods longer than six months, or in combination with prescription or illicit drugs. But, at present, there is no scientific data proving that consumption of ephedra/caffeine combinations for weight loss are unsafe, when consumed in accordance with appropriate warning labels. Additional research on the effects of ephedra on weight loss and in other areas, such as athletic performance, is clearly needed. I urge those who are responsible for policy to promote such research and to be guided by its findings.

Despite all the efforts to discredit her, Dr. Boozer's testimony earned a draw on the scorecard, more for her neutral and forthright position in a testimony brimming with agendas and politics.

Anti-Ephedra	17
Defended Ephedra	0
Draw	1

Unfortunately, additional research and studies were not in the cards at this time. Again, according to the *New York Times*, citing "several scientists [who] criticized studies paid for by the dietary supplements industry," said "given the possible dangers, it would now be unethical to ask anyone to take ephedra as part of a clinical trial."

There are two problems with this statement. The first questions of ephedra safety were raised a decade ago. Why didn't the NIH initiate any large-scale trials in that time? The NIH is comprised of twenty-seven separate components, mainly Institutes and Centers. It receives funding of $23,256,571,000 in Congressional appropriations. At present there are only two small-scale studies being conducted on ephedra, by the National Center for Complementary Medicine and Alternative

Health (and we already saw what they thought of ephedra with their "Consumer Alert" in Chapter 5.)

The second problem is that with the current massive tide of negativity against the herb, what scientist would be interested in putting together a grant proposal, especially if the attitude of "several scientists" is that it now would "be unethical to ask anyone to take ephedra as part of a clinical trial." What? Are we to believe no controversial pharmaceutical drugs are clinically tested?

Also appearing on the panel was Dr. Carlon M. Colker, M.D., Chief Executive Officer and Medical Director for Peak Wellness, Inc., in Greenwich, Connecticut. At first glance, Dr. Colker looked out of place on this panel, which could be loosely defined as the pro-ephedra panel—warts and all. You had all the company execs with some clouds in their past, plus Dr. Boozer, who endured more negative pre-publicity than anyone. Yet, here was Dr. Colker proudly defending ephedra.

During his testimony Dr. Colker said, "I have personally taken a variety of ephedra-based dietary supplements for the purpose of losing weight. I found that they worked well for me, over and above any adjustments to my diet and exercise. I also use ephedra-based products in my practice."

Dr. Colker's credentials seem impeccable; he is an attending physician at Beth Israel Medical Center in New York, as well as Greenwich Hospital in Connecticut. He was appointed by the State of Connecticut to the posts of Assistant Medical Examiner and Probate Court physician. He is also a fellow in the American College of Nutrition, and a member of the American College of Physicians and the American College of Sports Medicine, among many other professional medical organizations. There's one little problem with his resume—he accepted money from Cytodyne to perform a clinical evaluation of their ephedra product Xenadrine RFA-1. Another attempt at guilt by association? Is that what the panel designers were after? We're not sure, and no one will say.

Still, Dr. Colker was firmly in the pro-ephedra camp. Not

only that, he made recommendations the industry and government should be more interested in noting if public health is their overriding concern. Here's what Dr. Colker said: "While ephedra-based dietary supplements, including Xenadrine RFA-1, are appropriate for some people, there are populations for whom I think ephedra-based dietary supplements are not appropriate." Specifically, Dr. Colker mentioned people with contraindicated conditions—particularly without being monitored by their physician. He also said he believes there is significant abuse potential among youth and athletes. "Young people tend to fall into the scary mindset that 'more is better,'" said Dr. Colker. "Regulations should be designed accordingly to prevent sales to minors. Similarly, in general, athletes have a significant abuse potential in that some are willing to go to extremes to get an edge."

The defended ephedra team finally received a point, although it did rattle around the rim for a while.

Anti-Ephedra	17
Defended Ephedra	1
Draw	1

Panel Three managed to put only one other point in the "Defended Ephedra" column—that by the Major League Baseball Players Association. The rest of the testimonies were provided by sports organizations that already have banned ephedra, as well as Major League Baseball.

After tallying the results, the final score was:

Anti-Ephedra	23
Defended Ephedra	2
Draw	1

Oh, there was another potential point for the "Defended Ephedra" team that was ultimately withheld. This was a letter from forensic pathologist Dr. Michael Baden, former New York City chief medical examiner, who stated his opinion that the ephedra product taken by Orioles pitcher Steve Bechler very likely did not contribute to his death (see the beginning of Chapter 4 for entire quote). The letter was never read during the proceedings.

Two other speakers testified at the hearings: FDA Commissioner Mark B. McClellan, M.D., and Mr. J. Howard Beales III, Director of Bureau of Consumer Protection of the Federal Trade Commission (FTC). Dr. McClellan said once the agency finishes evaluating scientific data, probably later this summer, "we will take action." Whether that is likely to mean a ban on sales or new restrictions on the labels and marketing, is unclear. According to the *New York Times* account, "McClellan said the agency needs to make sure the evidence it is reviewing, such as studies on the herb and health complaints submitted to companies that use it in their products, could support a ban under the law. The 1994 statute requires the FDA to prove that a dietary supplement is harmful rather than having the manufacturer prove that it is safe, as with drugs."

It's very obvious that those who watched the hearings or read any accounts of them would come away with one unmistakable impression—ephedra is bad, bad, bad. But hey, I'm certain that was the desired outcome.

Chicken or Egg?

I finished up the hearing with the *New York Times* Dr. McClellan quote for a reason. It was only the last of many references during witnesses' testimony comparing drugs to dietary supplements; in particular, how unfair—and unsafe—the regulatory system is. It actually began with the *New York Times* article prior to the hearings, when the author's wrote, "While drug companies are required to prove the safety of their products and must turn over safety data and consumer complaints to the FDA, the agency, under a 1994 law, has no such authority over the makers of dietary supplements like ephedra." I'm not going to challenge these assertions until the next chapter, because I think there's something as important you should also know.

Remember this chapter's opening quote from Congressman Billy Tauzin? Perhaps the most telling aspect of his comments is when and where he made them. He didn't say this during the ephedra hearings, but rather at the time of the vote in the House on drug importations a few days later (I mentioned these in Chapter 5). Was Mr. Tauzin so moved by the testimony he heard, or was he trying to soften up the members of the House for a possible vote against ephedra and DSHEA?

It's impossible to tell whether companies, individuals or industries contribute funds to certain politicians because they already support their causes, or to nudge them to the contributor's way of thinking. Probably a better question is, does it really matter? Even if a member of Congress supports one particular piece of legislation favorable to an industry—for argument's sake, let's say the pharmaceutical industry—isn't that member of Congress likely to continue to support the industry's future positions as long as the dollars keep pouring in?

Let's look more closely at some aspects of Congress' relationships with the pharmaceutical and supplement industries First, here are the members of the Subcommittee on Oversight and Investigations, which was the key subcommittee for the July 2003 hearings "Issues Relating to Ephedra-containing Dietary Supplements."

Subcommittee Members
James C. Greenwood, Pennsylvania, Chairman
Michael Bilirakis, Florida
Cliff Stearns, Florida
Richard Burr, North Carolina

Charles F. Bass, New Hampshire
Greg Walden, Oregon, Vice Chairman
Mike Ferguson, New Jersey
Mike Rogers, Michigan
W.J. "Billy" Tauzin, Louisiana, (ex officio)
Peter Deutsch, Florida, Ranking Member
Diana DeGette, Colorado
Jim Davis, Florida
Jan Schakowsky, Illinois
Henry A. Waxman, California
Bobby L. Rush, Illinois
John D. Dingell, Michigan, (ex officio)

On the following pages are two lists; one shows the top recipients of pharmaceutical campaign contributions, and the other shows the top recipients of supplement industry contributions, with subcommittee members indicated with an asterisk (*). Five of the top seven members of the House of Representatives receiving campaign contributions from the pharmaceutical industry are on this subcommittee. One member of the subcommittee—Peter Deutsch—received contributions from dietary supplement companies.

Money talks, and you can definitely tell whose money is doing the talking here. Only one member of the House Subcommittee received money from the dietary supplement industry (and it was a measly $2,000), while six of the Subcommittee members received funds from the pharmaceutical industry, with those contributions ranging from approximately $66,000 to $130,000. Simply put, the supplement industry contributions amount to nothing more than chump change when compared to the drug dollars.

You might wonder why, in Chapter 5, I went off on a tangent and talked about the House of Representatives' vote on "Drug Importation" in August 2003, which received wide bipartisan support. According to the Center for Responsive Politics, cam-

Top Recipients of Political Donations within Pharmaceutical/Health Products Industry; Top 20 Members of the House; Election Cycle 2002

Rank	Candidate	Amount
1	Johnson, Nancy L (R-CT)	$211,317
*2	Dingell, John D (D-MI)	$130,498
*3	Tauzin, Billy (R-LA)	$119,750
*4	Ferguson, Mike (R-NJ)	$113,718
*5	Burr, Richard (R-NC)	$104,210
6	Thomas, Bill (R-CA)	$103,475
*7	Bilirakis, Michael (R-FL)	$95,742
8	Hastert, Dennis (R-IL)	$94,050
9	Blunt, Roy (R-MO)	$83,066
10	Sununu, John E (R-NH)	$82,999
11	Eshoo, Anna (D-CA)	$70,506
12	Bonilla, Henry (R-TX)	$67,845
13	Graham, Lindsey (R-SC)	$67,481
*14	Greenwood, James C (R-PA)	$66,475
15	Morella, Connie (R-MD)	$64,989
16	Upton, Fred (R-MI)	$64,424
17	Thune, John (R-SD)	$60,625
18	Ramstad, Jim (R-MN)	$60,401
19	Holt, Rush (D-NJ)	$58,361
20	Frelinghuysen, Rodney (R-NJ)	$58,113

Methlodogy: The numbers on this page are based on contributions from PACs and individuals giving $200 or more. All donations took place during the 2001–2002 election cycle and were released by the Federal Election Commission on Monday, April 28, 2003. Feel free to distribute or cite this material, but please credit the Center for Responsive Politics.

Top Recipients of Political Donations within Dietary Supplement Industry; Election Cycle 2002

Rank	Candidate	Amount
1	Istook, Ernest J (R-OK)	$37,000
2	Kennedy, Patrick J (D-RI)	$17,000
3	Burton, Dan (R-IN)	$9,000
4	Kucinich, Dennis J (D-OH)	$6,500
5	Pallone, Frank Jr (D-NJ)	$2,500
6	Thune, John (R-SD)	$2,000
*6	Deutsch, Peter (D-FL)	$2,000
6	Bonilla, Henry (R-TX)	$2,000
9	Morella, Connie (R-MD)	$1,000
9	Graham, Lindsey (R-SC)	$1,000
9	McInnis, Scott (R-CO)	$1,000
9	Lantos, Tom (D-CA)	$1,000
9	Cunningham, Randy (R-CA)	$1,000
9	Solis, Hilda L (D-CA)	$1,000
9	Phelps, David (D-IL)	$1,000
16	DeFazio, Peter (D-OR)	$500
16	Kolbe, Jim (R-AZ)	$500
18	Wu, David (D-OR)	$250

paign contribution figures show that lawmakers who sided with pharmaceutical interests (voting "no" on the bill) received an average of nearly three times the contributions from drug firms as those who took the alternate position (voting "yes"). Members who voted against the bill received an average of $39,813 in individual and PAC contributions from pharmaceutical manufacturers between 1989 and 2002. Members who voted for the bill received an average of $13,917 from the industry during that time.

The July 24, 2003 House vote on drug reimportation was unusual in that it did not break down along strict party lines, as many votes do. But the vote was not unusual in at least one major respect: campaign contributions were a solid indicator of the outcome.

The bill, which would ease the way for low-cost prescription drugs sold abroad to be "reimported" to the United States, passed by a vote of 243–186. Eighty-seven Republicans joined 155 Democrats and one Independent to support the bill in what represented a startling rebuke of the pharmaceutical industry, one of the most influential interests in Washington. Not surprisingly, the industry lobbied hard in opposing the bill.

Supporters of the bill say it would help to lower the cost of prescription drugs that are available at far cheaper prices abroad than they sell for domestically. The measure's opponents argue that reimported drugs could pose safety risks to consumers and hamper the innovation of new drugs.

It's interesting, if not helpful, to note how the Subcommittee on Oversight and Investigations—the subcommittee that conducted the July 2003 hearings regarding ephedra—voted on the bill. All six members on the above top-twenty list of contributions—Dingell, Tauzin, Ferguson, Burr, Bilirakis and Greenwood—voted "no" (in support of the pharmaceutical industry). Here's how the rest of the subcommittee members voted (the "yes" votes are noted with an asterisk *):

House Member	Vote	2001-2002 Contributions	1989-2002 Contributions
Stearns (R-FL)	N	$ 25,813	$81,613
DeGette (D-CO)	N	$12,503	$20,003
Waxman (D-CA)	N	$10,000	$87,850
Davis (D-FL)	N	$5,500	$10,567
Rogers (R-MI)	N	$7,000	$17,500
*Deutsch (D-FL)	Y	$5,000	$40,200
Rush (D-IL)	N	$3,500	$5,500

Walden (R-OR)	N	$3,500	$8,700
*Bass (R-NH)	Y	$500	$1,750
*Schakowsky (D-IL)	Y	$0	$0

Are these subcommittee members, who will largely be responsible for the fate of ephedra—and possibly DSHEA—"in bed" with the pharmaceutical industry? While it's difficult to prove definitively, the numbers certainly support the notion.

For the sake of argument, let's say that those who voted against the bill really could have had legitimate concerns with the bill, and thus voted "no." Well, let's look at what one of these representatives—Billy Tauzin (R-LA)—had to say about the issue:

Mr. Speaker, I join my colleague, the ranking member of our committee, the gentleman from Michigan (Mr. Dingell), in opposing this bill because it is dangerous.

And with this bill tonight, its authors I know are well-intentioned, angry at the price of drugs in America, angry at Canada because they impose price controls that take advantage of our citizens, angry at those trade laws that let it happen, they are asking us tonight to do exactly what we did in 1994—to vote for a bill that says safety does not matter when it comes to drugs, that safety does not really count; that we are going to repeal tonight, if they get their way, the language that is in the law that says that FDA must certify the safety of any drugs that are imported into this country; to take away the language that says FDA must do those things appropriate to ensure that the drug supply in this country is never compromised; that bogus, counterfeit, diluted, old, rotten drugs are not permitted into this country.

I voted wrong in 1994. I am not going to vote wrong tonight. I will never vote to compromise safety again in the use of drugs or products for our young people and our old people and our citizens.

Tonight we will learn about those rotten drugs that are coming into this country from Canada, yes, and from a lot of other countries, transhipped through Canada. We will have the smoking gun for tonight to show what is about to happen if we open the door to that awful problem.

Remember the two technologies I referred to in chapter 5 that could prevent counterfeiting—color-shifting dyes and a computer chip that prevents tampering with sealed packaging? Note that Mr. Tauzin makes no mention of them here. It's also kind of funny to see what lengths this guy will go to take shots at DSHEA and the supplement industry.

And what does PhRMA, the super-pharmaceutical lobby group, have to say on the issue? Here's a statement made by Alan F. Holmer, president of PhRMA: "To best benefit patients, Congress should focus on enacting Medicare drug coverage legislation and not on legislation dangerous to patients. The Gutknecht importation bill would jeopardize the safety of our nation's medicine supply and import foreign governments' price controls.

"However, we are pleased that a broadly bipartisan group of 53 Senators last night reiterated their strong opposition to changing current safety protection for patients. They urged the chairmen of the House-Senate Conference Committee to maintain the strong safety requirements pertaining to importation of drugs."

Hmmm, a lot of this language sounds awfully familiar, wouldn't you agree?

CHAPTER 10

Will Ephedra Destroy DSHEA?

"IN MY OPINION, the Dietary Supplement Health and Education Act (DSHEA) passed in 1994 has not provided a satisfactory framework to protect the public health by allowing dietary supplements to be marketed without prior approval of efficacy or safety by the FDA. Though DSHEA limits certain health claims for dietary supplements, these products are marketed in such a way that consumers believe they are effective to cure or treat many of the conditions that afflict the population, including obesity."

– Douglas Zipes, M.D., Distinguished Professor of Medicine Pharmacology and Toxicology Director of Division of Cardiology Krannert Institute of Cardiology, Indiana University School of Medicine in Indianapolis, in prepared testimony before the U.S. House Subcommittee on Oversight and Investigations Hearing, "Issues Relating to Ephedra-Containing Dietary Supplements," July 23–24, 2003

Is ephedra really the monster it's made out to be? Does it indeed kill large numbers of athletes, or result in innumerable cases of heart attack, stroke and other dangerous side effects? Or is the ephedra controversy simply a wedge issue—a ploy put forth by the pharmaceutical industry and others—designed to crack the door to DSHEA, enact tighter supplement controls, and ultimately destroy the dietary supplement industry? Maybe a lesson from ancient Greek mythology can provide a helpful illustration.

According to the well-known legend celebrated in the *Iliad* and the *Odyssey* of Homer, the Trojan horse was a huge, hollow wooden structure constructed by the Greeks to gain entrance into the city of Troy during the Trojan War in the 12th or 13th century B.C. In traditional accounts, Paris, son of the Trojan king, ran off with Helen, wife of Menelaus of Sparta, whose brother Agamemnon then led a Greek expedition against Troy. The ensuing war lasted ten years, finally ending when the Greeks pretended to be defeated and sailed to the nearby island of Tenedos to hide. Before doing so, they left behind a large wooden horse with a raiding party of armed warriors cleverly concealed inside. Sinon, a Greek who feigned desertion, convinced the Trojans that the horse was an offering to Athena that would make Troy impregnable.

Despite warnings of a devious plot, the Trojan horse was wheeled inside the city gates by the Trojans, who did not realize that Greek soldiers were hidden inside. That night, while the Trojans celebrated their victory, the Greeks snuck out of the wooden horse, opened the gates to their comrades—who had returned from Tenedos undiscovered—and succeeded in conquering Troy.

This brings us once again to the idea that perhaps the entire uproar is not about ephedra only. Could it instead be a sort of Trojan horse, employed by the drug industry and others to gain access to the fort surrounding DSHEA? If this is a plot with designs that extend beyond pubic safety, then shame on the perpetrators in hiding. I'm sure everyone agrees the public deserves safe and effective dietary supplement products. However, they also ought to have straightforward, balanced, and responsible reporting by both the media and government on the safety and benefits of these products.

Dastardly DSHEA

When attacking DSHEA and the supplement industry, critics usually cite variations of one of two themes: 1) At best, supplements don't do anything but waste people's money. And at worst, they can harm—or even kill—you. 2) Government regulators are powerless to regulate supplements under DSHEA.

To show how this first issue works—apart from ephedra—let's look at a study appearing in the April 10, 2002 issue of the *Journal of the American Medical Association.* In that issue, *JAMA* published the results of the NIH's first large-scale trial on St. John's wort (*Hypericum perforatum*) and depression. You might remember the news accounts generated from the study, which didn't vary much from a headline appearing on a press release from the National Institute of Mental Health (NIHM): "Study Shows St. John's Wort Ineffective for Major Depression of Moderate Severity."

There are a few things of interest here. First, on the bottle of St. John's wort (SJW) I take, it says it is for "mood enhancement," not necessarily moderate depression. I find when I'm under stress, it helps take the edge off and my focus improves.

But here's the most interesting finding of the study. It found that neither SJW nor the prescription drug Zoloft (sertraline) were more effective than placebo in this particular trial. Media coverage fixed solely on SJW, erroneously reporting that "St. John's wort doesn't work," yet they did not even mention Zoloft's ineffectiveness. Just to be sure, here is what the authors stated in the abstract of their study: "Interventions patients were randomly assigned to receive *H. perforatum*, placebo, or sertraline (as an active comparator) for eight weeks. Based on clinical response, the daily dose of *H. perforatum* could range from 900 to 1,500 mg and that of sertraline from 50 to 100 mg. Responders at week eight could continue blinded treatment for another eighteen weeks.

"Results on the two primary outcome measures, *neither sertraline [Zoloft] nor* H. perforatum *was significantly different from placebo."*

And what did NIMH say about the study? "The multi-site trial, involving 340 participants, also compared the FDA-approved antidepressant drug sertraline (Zoloft) to placebo as a way to measure how sensitive the trial was to detecting antidepressant effects."

It continued, "The trial . . . was launched in response to the growing use of St. John's wort in the United States and a need for more definitive data on its use for different types of depression. Although several smaller European studies have suggested that St. John's wort is useful in treating mild to moderately severe depression, experts who reviewed those studies concluded that they had limitations and more rigorous trials were needed before firm conclusions could be drawn."

You then have to traverse five dense paragraphs about SJW and depression before you reach this (emphasis is mine): "The overall response to sertraline on the primary measures was not superior to that of placebo, an outcome which is not uncommon in trials of approved antidepressants. *In fact, this apparent lack of efficacy occurs in up to 35 percent of trials of antidepressants."*

Did I miss something? Why didn't the article writers investigate more closely why Zoloft, which is marketed for depression and which costs far more than St. John's wort, didn't perform better? I think the real story here is that if this study is any indicator of truth, it demonstrates that a drug, with sales of over $2 billion and prescribed to millions of Americans for severe forms of depression, may be no more effective than placebo. Zoloft costs around $100 for thirty pills, St. John's wort ranges between a few to several dollars for a month's supply, and a placebo costs virtually nothing! Again, shouldn't the news report have at least mentioned this?

Perspectives on DSHEA

In the early 1990s, Congress examined ways to battle health frauds including nutritional or therapeutic claims. During the same period, the FDA was considering tighter regulations for supplement labels.

In response, the health-food industry urged Congress to "preserve the consumer's freedom to choose dietary supplements" and warned retailers that the regulations under consideration would cripple their business. Consumers were told that unless they took action, the FDA would take away their right to buy vitamins. As a result, Congress received piles of letters from concerned citizens.

According to a 1997 article appearing in *PR Watch,* which is published by the Center for Media & Democracy, in 1992 supplement makers called on the Rogers & Cowan PR firm to help launch the Nutritional Health Alliance, a grassroots PR campaign aimed at fighting what it called "the FDA's bias against preventive medicine and the dietary supplement industry."

Under the FDA's proposed rules for implementing its powers, supplements marketed simply as nutritional aids would be subject to the same rules as other food products, while substances marketed as disease cures or treatments would be held to the same "safety and efficacy" standard as drugs sold by the pharmaceutical industry.

According to *PR Watch,* one TV advertisement depicted mock FDA agents dressed in riot gear, who raided Mel Gibson's house and confiscated his vitamins. Gibson joined celebrities such as Whoopi Goldberg, Randy Travis, Sissy Spacek, Laura Dern, Mariel Hemingway and Victoria Principal in making public service announcements claiming that the FDA was trying to block consumer access to vitamins.

Vitamin sellers, along with ten thousand health food stores and their customers, supported the movement by targeted advertising and flyers calling on supporters to "act now to protect your right to use safe vitamins, minerals, herbs, and other dietary supplements of your choice." One brochure by the NHA urged consumers to "write to Congress today or kiss your supplements goodbye."

PR Watch says the goal of the campaign was to ensure passage of DSHEA, a bill sponsored by Utah Senator Orrin S. Hatch. Displays were set up at health food stores with copies of letters to be sent to members of Congress. Some stores offered discounts to participants. Others provided free phone lines to call lawmakers. During a nationwide "blackout day," stores refused to sell products that they claimed were threatened. NHA's director warned darkly of a "worldwide conspiracy" led by the "pharmaceutical-medical combine trying to make sure they are not being threatened worldwide by inexpensive, non-patented dietary supplements that will prevent the onset of chronic disease." In the space of twelve months, the campaign generated more than one hundred thousand letters to members of Congress, more than half of whom eventually agreed to cosponsor the legislation.

Bruce Silverglade, director of legal affairs for the Center for Science in the Public Interest, said the campaign was a "big lie." "The consumers who wrote Congress had a financial interest in the matter or were duped into believing the FDA was using the new labeling law to ban their favorite vitamins. . . . People should have the right to try any type of health care that they choose. But what we're talking about is whether the manufacturers have the right to hype supplements on the basis of unreliable scientific information or downright false claims."

The end result was passage of DSHEA, which defined "dietary supplements" as a separate regulatory category. DSHEA also created an NIH Office of Dietary Supplements and directed the President to appoint a Commission on Dietary Supplement Labels to recommend ways to implement the act.

The Commission's final recommendations were released on November 24, 1997.

Of Primrose and Black Currant Oil

Here's another view of how DSHEA came about; this one from Stephen N. McNamara and A. Wes Siegner, Jr. Partners at the law firm Hyman, Phelps & McNamara, P.C. in Washington, D.C.

"DSHEA was enacted because FDA was viewed as distorting the law that existed before DSHEA to try improperly to deprive the public of safe and popular dietary supplement products," they wrote in an article appearing in the journal produced by the Food and Drug Law Institute. After abusing its powers regarding dietary supplements, the "FDA's authority needed to be better defined and controlled." Although Mr. Siegner is known as someone who has defended ephedra on occasion, the law firm assists the drug industry with respect to the regulation of foods, drugs, medical devices, cosmetics, and related products. The firm's clients include companies that manufacture and distribute both dietary supplements and pharmaceutical drugs.

The attorneys say DSHEA was passed by unanimous consent because of abuse of power by the FDA. They provide two examples of FDA excesses described by a Senate Committee. One was the FDA campaign to prevent the marketing of dietary supplements of black currant oil (from the same fruit used to make jam). The FDA argued the addition of black currant oil to a gelatin capsule caused the black currant oil to become a "food additive" as defined by FDCA, and that as a "food additive," the substance could not be marketed as a dietary supplement without first obtaining FDA issuance of an approving "food additive" regulation. Typically, the Senate noted, "the cost to a manufacturer to prepare a food additive petition can run to $2 million. FDA approval of a food additive petition typically takes from two to six years."

In case you're curious, black currant oil differs from other essential fatty acid oils because it contains both omega-6 gamma-linolenic acid and omega-3 alpha linolenic acid. It's believed to support the body's manufacture of hormone-like substances known as prostaglandins, which help regulate functions of the circulatory system.

After the Seventh Circuit Court ruled against the FDA, the U.S. Court of Appeals for the First Circuit, ruled similarly, saying that the "FDA's reading of the Act is nonsensical. . . . The proposition that placing a single-ingredient food product into an inert capsule as a convenient method of ingestion converts that food into a food additive perverts the statutory text, undermines legislative intent, and defenestrates common sense. We cannot accept such anfractuous reasoning."

A similar thing happened regarding the FDA's attempts to ban another dietary supplement; evening primrose oil. (In England, it is an approved treatment for breast pain and allergic dermatitis and eczema.) Although evening primrose oil was considered to be a safe and popular dietary supplement, the FDA claimed it, too, was an "unapproved food additive." These two rulings against the FDA helped pave the way for passage of DSHEA.

As an illustration of the agency's organized effort to undermine certain dietary supplements, evidence was presented before the House of Representatives and the Senate in 1993 that the FDA Commissioner had awarded the Commissioner's Special Citation to more than FDA personnel, who at that time comprised the "Evening Primrose Oil Litigation Team." Nevertheless, although two U.S. district courts and two three-judge U.S. courts of appeals had all unanimously rejected FDA's regulatory program, Congress concluded that unless it stepped in and passed DSHEA, the facts showed that FDA would continue to try to prohibit the marketing of safe and proper dietary supplements. In the hearing on "Dietary Supplements," Before the House Committee on Appropriations, Subcommittee on

Agriculture, Rural Development, Food and Drug Administration, and Related Agencies, in October 1993, the committee wrote, "The committee is therefore concerned that the FDA will persist in such litigation, and thereby continue to subject small manufacturers to the choice of abandoning production and sale of lawful products, or accepting the significant financial burden of defending themselves against baseless lawsuits brought by the FDA."

McNamara and Siegner say it is important to remember this history, both because it helps to explain why, under current law, the FDA is not entrusted with blanket pre-approval authority over the marketing of all dietary supplement products, and because "it illustrates the risk of excessively-restrictive regulation that might be presented if FDA were to be given such comprehensive preclearance authority in the future.

Getting Around the Act

The Food, Drug, and Cosmetic Act defines "drug" as any article (except devices) "intended for use in the diagnosis, cure, mitigation, treatment, or prevention of disease" and "articles (other than food) intended to affect the structure or function of the body." These words permit the FDA to stop the marketing of products with unsubstantiated "drug" claims on their labels.

According to Stephen Barrett, M.D., of Quackwatch, to get around the intent of the law, the supplement industry has deviously sought ways to promote "medicinal" uses to the public that are not stated on product labels. This is done mainly by promoting the ingredients of the products through a variety of channels such as books, magazines, newsletters, booklets, lectures, and radio and television broadcasts and on the Internet.

"DSHEA worsened this situation by increasing the amount of misinformation that can be directly transmitted to prospective customers," said Barrett. "It also expanded the types of products that could be marketed as 'supplements.' Although many such products—particularly herbs—are marketed for their alleged preventive or therapeutic effects," he added, "the 1994 law has made it difficult or impossible for the FDA to regulate them as drugs." Actually they can, as you'll see below.

Here's another viewpoint. According to the Institute of Food Technologists' IFT's Summary, published in the July 1999 issue of *Food Technology*, this act broadened the definition of supplements to include ingredients not recognized as traditional nutrients, such as botanicals and hormones.

"Prior to DSHEA, these ingredients could have been challenged by the FDA as unapproved food additives, [but they are now] exempt from additive regulations applicable to conventional foods," note summary authors Mary Ellen Camire, Ph.D., University of Maine, and Mark A. Kantor, Ph.D., University of Maryland.

Although supplement manufacturers should ensure that their products are safe and be able to provide information to support any labeling claims, the FDA bears the burden of showing that a supplement is unsafe or mislabeled before it can restrict or ban the product's use, say Camire and Kantor. "The passage of DSHEA has created an economic and regulatory environment favorable to the expanded marketing, sales, and distribution of dietary supplements," they note. "Opportunities for consumers to purchase supplements in a free market economy are vastly increased, but [false] expectations remain that government agencies provide [consumer] protection from unsafe or mislabeled products. One of the future challenges with respect to supplements will be to reconcile these apparently opposing forces."

The Truth About DSHEA and Ephedra

According to McNamara and Siegner, the FDA already has the power to regulate any dietary supplement under DSHEA. If the FDA claims that ephedra is unsafe, or violates any of the following conditions, it can remove it.

A dietary supplement that is "adulterated" or "misbranded," or that bears an unauthorized drug claim is subject to seizure, condemnation and destruction. DSHEA included additional safety requirements regarding the introduction of new dietary ingredients. The law clarified that dietary supplement ingredients marketed prior to October 15, 1994 do not require pre-market approval. However, manufacturers marketing a new dietary supplement ingredient after this date must submit safety information on the new dietary ingredient to FDA.

Also DSHEA provides the Secretary of Health and Human Services with the authority to remove *any* dietary supplement or dietary supplement ingredient that poses an "imminent hazard." If the HHS Secretary makes this decision, the government must conduct an administrative review of the case and the product cannot be sold to the public. In addition, the FTC also has the ability to remove products and punish companies guilty of fraudulent advertising and promotion.

Going back to Chapter 3, the FDA can remove products from the market for the following reasons:

Misleading Labeling/Failure to Warn: According to the FDA, many makers of dietary supplements containing ephedra are selling products containing significantly less—or much more—ephedra than stated on the label, according to a study published in the *American Journal of Health-System Pharmacy*. Some times, consumers have no way of telling how much ephedrine they are ingesting with each tablet. If that's the case, the FDA has to power to remove these products.

Poses A Significant and Unreasonable Risk: The FDA does not have to prove that a product actually harmed anyone, but simply that it presents a "significant or unreasonable risk" of illness or injury. Does the scientific evidence on the safety and efficacy of ephedra's consumption show that it poses a significant or unreasonable risk? Not the studies I've seen.

On the other hand, there are people who die every year from violent allergic reactions to common foods such as peanuts and shellfish. So should we ban peanuts and shellfish? Of course not. And that's because relatively few people are adversely affected (and since I live in Georgia I know peanut farmers would storm Washington, D.C.!)

Contains Poisonous or Deleterious Substances: The FDA does not have to prove that a ephedra product has a substance that will injure, but simply that it *may* render injury under the recommended or suggested conditions indicated on a product's label. Studies show that ephedra dietary supplements, when used according to industry standards are safe for most people. Perfect for everyone? By no means.

Is Unfit for Food: Although technically ephedra is not considered a "food," the FDA has authority to stop the marketing of any dietary supplement that the agency believes is not fit for human consumption. There is no evidence whatsoever that ephedra is unfit for human consumption.

Makes Drug Claims: If a dietary supplement's label indicates that the product can diagnose, cure, mitigate, treat or prevent a disease, then it is clearly being represented as a "drug" and is no longer considered a dietary supplement. Responsible manufacturers have labels, warnings, and directions for use for their products and do not represent their products as drugs.

Lacks Truthful and Informative Labeling: By law, all dietary supplement products must contain extensive informative labeling, including detailed information about the nutrients in the product, such as name and quantity of all ingredients in the product and the name and place of business of the company, for example. Industry supports enforcement efforts of this provision. Recently the Secretary of Health and Human Services announced enforcement efforts to remove products that were marketed to minors and for illicit purposes. The dietary supplement industry has consistently urged the FDA to use its enforcement powers to remove such products from the marketplace.

There are other protections as well. The FTC monitors false advertising and also has the power to shut down fraudulent operations. Magazines, newspapers and broadcast outlets also have a code of ethics against false or misleading advertising. Are these enforced? Of course not. I'm sure plenty of us have been suckered into buying a device that comes with the guarantee of being able to see through walls—or a magic pill that can solve a myriad of health problems. But the simple truth is that the power to ban these items exists.

So, the FDA, the Department of Health and Human Services, and the FTC all have broad powers to remove any product that is an "imminent hazard," "deleterious," "a significant risk," and so on. This begs the question: Why haven't they done so with ephedra before now? Considering all the facts contained in this book (and a lot more that couldn't be discussed), we should all ask ourselves what is going on with ephedra. According to Metabolife company records supplied to HHS, over the last five years more than 4.5 billion tablets and 50 million bottles of Metabolife 356 have been sold. The company also claimed it recorded 14,700 "incident reports," with about 78 of the reports appearing to be serious incidents, including hospitalizations and reportedly one death. According to some experts who have reviewed them, this level of adverse incidents is consistent with the occurrence of these conditions in the general population. That means that people taking 4.5 billion placebo or sugar pills would report just as many "incident reports."

There's also a risk of misinterpretation of data or overreaction to misread data. When Metabolife released its record of

AERs, various media accounts stated that all 14,700 "incident reports" were "serious"—clearly a gross exaggeration. Where did they get this information from? They didn't make it up.

But that is probably beyond the point. Many experts, including the GAO and the FDA, now say AERs are not a valid scientific basis upon which to develop regulatory policy on the safety of a substance. But, when the average consumer reads these numbers as fact, the information resonates.

How's This for Irony?

The DSHEA is often portrayed as the wild teenager running amok under the blind eye of mother FDA, causing unbelievable angst among its food and drug siblings. Then, as I wrote this chapter, two things occurred that made DSHEA seem more like the unloved stepchild and the food and drug siblings like the sneaky kids committing dreadful acts out behind the barn. One of these things was the creation of the new label law for the fat substitute olestra, and the other was the release of a study focusing on the popular antidepressant Paxil and its role in suicidal behavior in children.

In August 2003, the FDA ruled that snack foods made with the zero-calorie fat substitute olestra no longer had to bear the label warning stating that it can cause cramps and diarrhea. The FDA said it was allowing Procter & Gamble to remove the warning since research showed that any stomach-troubling effect is mild and rare.

The FDA approved olestra's sale in 1996, but with labels detailing possible gastrointestinal side effects. The synthetic chemical made of sugar and soybeans tastes like fat, but passes through the body undigested. It is believed the warning limited sales of the products (possibly by party hosts fearful of embarrassing incidents?). P&G argued the fake fat was safe and the complaints unfair, since stomach upset and diarrhea are common anyway.

The FDA said it was swayed by a study that tracked how 3,000 people felt after eating chips during a six-week period. Half ate chips with olestra, and half ate chips they thought contained olestra but really didn't. The study showed olestra eaters had only slightly more frequent bowel movements than the people who ate full-fat chips.

The Center for Science in the Public Interest (CSPI) disagreed vehemently with the FDA's decisions. Last year, it said the FDA had close to *twenty thousand* reports of problems and the FDA has logged more complaints about olestra than it has about all other food additives in history combined. In a press release entitled, "FDA Caves in on Olestra," CSPI said the FDA gave into the wishes of P&G, and "without an adequate warning label, olestra-containing chips may inadvertently find their way into shopping carts and lunchboxes of even those consumers who are trying to avoid olestra."

Now, to that Paxil study. On August 5, 2003, the *Boston Globe* reported on a growing body of evidence linking Paxil, made by GlaxoSmithKline, to suicidal thoughts and actions in a small percentage of the children who take it. In June, the FDA recommended that doctors stop prescribing Paxil to new patients under the age of eighteen and advised parents to consult a doctor if their children are currently taking Paxil. Notice the FDA only "recommends" that parents talk to their child's doctor.

According to the *Globe* account, not long before the FDA's announcement, its British counterpart took a strong stance against Paxil, advising doctors not to prescribe it to children after reviewing clinical trial data of about 1,000 children on the drug who had a one-and-a-half to three times greater risk of having suicidal thoughts than those taking placebos. But the FDA is more vague about its plans, waiting to deliver the final word on Paxil while it reviews the data. The *Globe* story quotes Mary Anne Rhyne, a spokeswoman for GlaxoSmithKline as saying that the number of children on Paxil who experience suicidal thoughts is "a relatively small number of patients. We think there is more research that needs to be done."

There are two extremely intriguing—if not provocative—statements contained in the FDA's press release regarding the problems. First there's this warning: "Advisory: Despite the new possible safety concerns about use of Paxil in children, it is essential that patients taking Paxil (paroxetine hydrochloride) do not suddenly discontinue use of the drug. Any changes must take place under medical supervision."

The advisory is followed by this statement: "Three well-controlled trials in pediatric patients with MDD [major depressive disorder] failed to show that the drug was more effective than placebo. The new safety information that is currently under review was derived from trials of Paxil in pediatric patients."

In other words, even though we realize that Paxil doesn't work, please continue to take it, especially since your doctor prescribed it.

Presently, Prozac is the only antidepressant approved for children, with studies demonstrating its effectiveness in young people. But even without approval, a drug like Paxil can still be prescribed to children. Once the FDA approves a drug for a certain group of patients with a particular condition, doctors are free to prescribe it to whomever they feel might benefit, including children and individuals with conditions the FDA did not consider. What makes this even more alarming is that we're talking about children—people who are either too young, not responsible for their own health-care decisions, or both—that are taking this drug.

I have one question—why on earth wasn't this possible risk publicized more widely? I can only imagine the headlines if the subject of this story were ephedra—or any dietary supplement for that matter—and its potential link with teen suicide.

What Does the Future Hold?

As with any controversy, there are plenty of rumors. There's no question that important facets of DSHEA have never been implemented and enforced. Some Washington insiders say FDA staffers have admitted, off the record, that they have not been forthcoming with regulations such as Good Manufacturing Practices (GMPs)—as DSHEA required the FDA to do eight years ago—because they wanted to create an issue that would result in rewriting DSHEA.

Some think the ephedra issue is part of a larger plan to not only undermine DSHEA, but also to join a worldwide movement that would essentially destroy the dietary supplement industry. Seem too much like a "conspiracy theory" sort of statement? Maybe, but consider this. There exists an organization, called the Codex Alimentarius, which is a United Nations commission that is also part of the World Health Organization. The goal of the Codex Alimentarius Commission is to set international standards for anything consumed by humans. For dietary supplement products, the intent is to establish an international guideline stating that no supplements can be sold for preventive or therapeutic purposes. No problem there—such a guideline already exists under DSHEA.

But here is where it gets scary. The Codex Alimentarius Commission also wants to limit over-the-counter sales of dietary supplements to potencies consistent with the Recommended Dietary Allowance (RDA) levels, which are set to merely to prevent deficiencies and the conditions—such as beri-beri or scurvy—that result from those deficiencies. Any product that contains higher levels of vitamins, minerals or other ingredients—such as your daily multivitamin or the bottle of vitamin C on the grocery store shelf—would theoretically become pharmaceuticals. In other words, you would probably need a prescription to get a daily multivitamin.

Who would be behind this? Take a wild guess. Here's what

well-known dietary consultant and author Gary Null wrote about the Codex Alimentarius Commission in the September 1999 issue of *Penthouse*: "In recent years . . . big medicine, the pharmaceutical establishment, and their allies in big government all joined forces to protect their own interests. These threatened groups engage in fear-mongering before Congress to get legislation that would sic state medical boards on alternative therapies, let dietitians control the dispensing of nutritional advice, and keep the public from having freedom of choice by turning as many nutrients as possible into prescription drugs. This is what the future will bring unless we take action."

He continues, "Not far into the twenty-first century you may be saying so long to your St. John's wort, goodbye to your *Ginkgo biloba*. These and many other supplements may become things of the past, at least as reasonably priced over-the-counter items."

Paranoia? Perhaps. But as a friend once told me, "Just because you're paranoid doesn't mean people aren't out to get you."

CHAPTER 11

Conclusion: What Happens Next?

"OBVIOUSLY, IT IS very important that the FDA has an accurate and effective system. People's lives may depend on it. Companies' reputations are at stake. Sometimes millions or billions of dollars of investments can be affected. So it is very important that the FDA does a good job in this area."

– Opening remarks of Chairman Dan Burton (R-IN), Hearing before the Committee on Government Reform, House of Representatives, May 27, 1999; "How Accurate is the FDA's Monitoring of Supplements Like Ephedra?"

By the time you read this, ephedra could be no more, at least as a widely available over-the-counter supplement. And that would be unfortunate. I say that not because I'm a big fan or because I know it is 100 percent safe. I don't know that, and neither does anyone else. And therein lies the rub. The problem is, we don't truly know its risks (and if it does have risks, how severe they are). The number of deaths attributed to it vary from a very few to over one hundred. And interpretations of the existing data concerning ephedra, including that contained in the RAND report, are all over the map. It's as if the report was compiled by Rand-McNally.

There is a basic marketing axiom that says if you repeat a statement often enough, people will accept it as truth. And it's even more believable if you can get someone else to say it. In ephedra's case, if you say it is dangerous—or even better, if you can get the media to say it is dangerous—many, many people will simply believe it.

The same can be said for DSHEA. If people continuously read and hear that dietary supplements are unregulated and/or dangerous and that the FDA's hands are tied, making it unable to exert any authority on the industry, people will believe it. And if people accept that both ephedra and DSHEA put the public's health at risk, the message resonates even more.

Let's Talk about Public Health

The notion that public health is at risk is supposed to be the overriding factor in the apparent movement to do away with ephedra and DSHEA. Frankly, this notion should be at the top of the list of any discussion regarding things we put in our bodies, whether it's food, prescription or OTC drugs, or dietary supplements. No doubt there are phony print ads and TV infomercials hyping "natural" supplements for bigger breasts and smaller thighs, weight loss, muscle gain, hair restoration and longer life. While they all sound too good to be true, we want to believe that they're accurate; we want to trust that the FDA and other regulatory agencies are on top of these things; we want to assume that if it's on the store shelf, then it must be safe. The truth is, sometimes these products are, but sometimes they aren't. And supplements containing ephedra alkaloids and other substances are no exception.

Have some of the companies selling ephedra made exaggerated claims, tried to manipulate studies, or held back important information? I'm sure they have. And those that have been caught are being punished, as they should be. It seems, though, that we only hear about the bad ones.

Let's not be naïve and think that this is something that occurs only with ephedra companies. Any time there is a profit motive, or the opposite, a fear of monetary loss, unscrupulous people will try to tweak—or outright alter—the results. That goes for any product, whether it be dietary supplements, pharmaceutical drugs, baby carriages, or garden hoses.

If public health is assumed to be the number-one concern, here are a few questions I'd like to have answered by the FDA:

- Why hasn't the FDA—and the NIH—pushed for more large-scale tests on ephedra and other supplements over the past decade?
- How many people have died as a direct result of taking ephedra? One, five, thirty, "dozens," one hundred, five hundred? When reporters get it wrong, why doesn't the FDA correct them?
- When will the FDA publicize all the thousands of deaths and injuries from prescription and OTC drugs with the same shrill alarm as it has with ephedra?
- Why doesn't the FDA speak out more about the safety record of pharmaceuticals with the same vigor it does with dietary supplements?
- How about recalls? Despite no formal manufacturing standards for supplements, according to the *Federal Register* from March 13, 2003, the FDA received reports on an average of twenty dietary supplement recalls per year from 1990 to 1999. I'm curious—how does that stack up against pharmaceutical drugs?
- Why, since the inception of DSHEA, has the FDA failed to implement every aspect of the Act required under the law?

There is supposed to be a Dietary Supplement Strategy Ten-Year Plan. Is this plan on track? If not, why? Is it a funding problem? Or has it simply been ignored?

The truth is, ephedra has never been adequately tested. The relatively few trials investigating its weight loss and athletic endurance capabilities were small and focused on short-term effects. For some strange reason, the NIH has never sponsored a major, large-scale trial over the past decade (the NIH houses the Office of Dietary Supplements, whose mission is to expand research and provide consumer information about dietary supplements). It seems there has been more research devoted to discrediting the herb than to determining if it's effective and/or safe.

Those opposed to ephedra and DSHEA say—at least privately—that there is an unfair advantage since products under DSHEA have never had to pass the regulatory muster and undergo the expense prescription drugs endure. What they fail to acknowledge though, is a large chunk of the research on prescription drugs is essentially carried out gratis, free, complements of the National Institutes of Health. They also fail to acknowledge that undertaking the FDA approval process essentially guarantees a patent on the drug, which allows for years of possessing a corner on the market and the potential to amass millions—even billions—of dollars in return. Finally, you'll rarely hear these folks mention that, unlike FDA-approved drugs, supplements are extremely limited in the health claims their labels can feature.

Stephen N. McNamara and A. Wes Siegner, Jr. (partners at the law firm of Hyman, Phelps & McNamara, P.C. in Washington, D.C.) say that the favorite argument of the FDA and the media—namely, that the FDA has little or no authority to regulate the supplement industry—is bogus. Rather, McNamara and Siegner, Jr. believe that the FDA has not exercised the full extent of its authority. In an article they authored in a 2002 issue of the journal produced by the Food and Drug Law Institute entitled, "FDA Has Substantial and Sufficient Authority to Regulate Dietary Supplements," they wrote, "FDA's existing powers are substantial and are more than sufficient for the agency to regulate dietary supplements successfully for the protection of the public health. There is no need to amend DSHEA to increase FDA's authority over such products."

Here's another example. In an announcement issued on September 23, 1997 in the *Federal Register*, the FDA stated that current law requires all dietary supplement products to contain 100 percent of the labeled amount of each added dietary ingredient for the entire shelf life of the supplement. Despite this, the agency has not made any sustained effort to follow up, investigate, and take regulatory actions against dietary supplement products that have been identified in the media as not containing the full amount of the ingredients declared on their labels. "The FDA has ample authority to act against supplements that do not provide the full amounts of the nutrients they are labeled as providing," said McNamara and Siegner. "Yet the agency has done almost nothing to use this authority."

If Ephedra Survives

Let's assume that somehow ephedra survives and the government doesn't ban it. What should be done? What promises and commitments must manufacturers and distributors of ephedra products make; and conversely, what should be required of the regulatory government agencies?

The government could take the easy (some would say cowardly) way out by reducing the daily dosage size of ephedra to the levels it recommended in 1997. If the agency does that, many experts believe that the herb is as good as gone. At those low levels few people, if any, would experience any benefit and would therefore stop using it.

Instead, the FDA needs to do four things, keeping as its top priority one thing—that of the public's health.

1. *Immediately arrange for the NIH to initiate at least one (if not many) large-scale, double-blind, placebo-controlled study.* As many an expert has said, though the preliminary data we have seems to indicate that ephedra is not the killer herb many make it out to be, large-scale, double-blind trials will go a long way in demonstrating for certain whether ephedra is safe and/or effective as a dietary supplement.

2. *Finalize Good Manufacturing Practices (GMPs or CGMPs) setting requirements for potency, purity, sanitary conditions and record keeping.* This has been promised for over eight years, and the longer the FDA waits, the more it jeopardizes public health. Also, DSHEA requires manufacturers submit adequate information on the safety of any new ingredients contained in dietary supplements before they can be sold.

It's easy to get the impression that the dietary supplement industry has dragged its feet; that somehow it is to their advantage to have shoddy, dangerous products on the market. Here's a little nugget of truth, found in the FDA's own documents: "On November 20, 1995, representatives of the dietary supplement industry submitted to FDA an outline for CGMP regulations for dietary supplements and dietary supplement ingredients. We evaluated the outline and determined that it provided a useful starting point for developing CGMP regulations. Nonetheless, we believed that the industry outline did not address certain issues that should be considered when developing a proposed rule on CGMPs for dietary ingredients and dietary supplements. For example, the industry outline did not address the need for specific controls for automatic, computer-controlled or assisted systems." That was nearly eight years ago.

In March of 2003, the FDA proposed new CGMP guidelines

for supplements. Isn't it in the best interest of public safety to make such guidelines official as soon as possible?

3. *Develop an Adverse Reaction Reporting System for all FDA products.* If public health is the number-one concern, no product—be it bad bread, an herb or an OTC medication—should be excluded from the database. Whenever ephedra critics bring up AERs for ephedra, the public is never told that there is no general requirement for the reporting of adverse experiences to FDA, even for nonprescription (over-the-counter) drug products. "There would appear to be little reason," write McNamara and Siegner, "why a mandatory adverse experience reporting system and a government bureaucracy to manage the system should be established for dietary supplements, such as tablets of vitamin C, when such requirements do not apply to aspirin or other nonprescription drugs." I agree. If we are to have a reporting system for one industry, we should have such a system for all the industries under the FDA's umbrella.

4. *Call a legitimate summit of experts.* I have yet to see an industry that effectively polices itself. There may be such a thing, but I doubt it. That is why we have laws and "unbiased" regulatory agencies. But these laws must have teeth, and the lawmakers must approve the necessary funds so the regulators can do their jobs. Additionally, it is crucial that the regulators perform their duties without undue influence from those they are regulating. Otherwise, public safety is ultimately jeopardized.

Thus, the HHS and FDA need to organize an "ephedra summit," to which they would invite scientists, health and fitness experts, lawmakers and manufacturers to come and hash out a standards for the production, distribution and consumption of ephedra. These standards, of course, should be based on the latest legitimate data (and if future studies prove the standards need to be changed, the FDA should allow for this to occur in an expedient manner). Scientists working on behalf of the

Ephedra Education Council already have formalized a list of suggested "National Standards." This list might be a good starting point.

In order for this summit to achieve its purpose, politics would have to be checked at the door. Anyone who is receiving or has received campaign contributions from either pharmaceutical companies or dietary supplement companies would have to reveal that fact in the public record. The same goes for any honorariums that scientists have received. (Ideally these people would be excluded altogether, but it's doubtful that could be accomplished.) Simply put, there is no place for political or financial conflict of interest in this process.

In the summer of 2002, the National Academy of Science's Institute of Medicine released a 156-page draft report on its framework to evaluate the safety of dietary supplements. If adopted by the FDA, it could help establish a (hopefully) rational system to determine safety of popular supplement ingredients.

Is It Too Late?

I've said this before, but it bears repeating: If ephedra is so dangerous, so risky, why hasn't the FDA or HHS yanked it from the shelves? After all, they have the authority to do just that. Senator Dick Durbin (D-IL), who chaired a hearing on weight-loss supplements, called on HHS Secretary Tommy Thompson to determine immediately whether ephedra supplements pose an "imminent hazard" to public health, and if so, to suspend sales of such products. He is also sponsoring a bill, S.722 ("Dietary Supplement Safety Act"), which, if passed, could greatly alter or even do away with DSHEA.

The cynic in me thinks that as long as ephedra stays in the news, the easier it will be to link it to the movement against DSHEA. That way, the FDA could eliminate both in one fell swoop. I hope my cynicism is misplaced. With numerous special interest groups—most wielding substantial financial and/or political power—lining up against it, along with a public swayed by misguided media reports, it might be too late for ephedra. Hopefully, it's not too late for the rest of the supplement industry.

Afterword: Author's Note

While writing this book, I have gone against much popular thought and opinion and questioned many powerful government agencies, officials, industries, and professions. I have taken stands contrary to organizations I often listen to and respect, such as the Center for Science in the Public Interest and Public Citizen. While conducting my research, I often asked myself "Am I sure I'm right?" At times it shook my confidence, but then I stumbled upon something else that made no sense or was flat-out wrong. When that happened I pushed on . . .

I'd also like to thank the people at Woodland Publishing for allowing me to develop this book as I saw fit. Once I began, they graciously stepped out of the way. Although they might have cringed at times at things I uncovered, I suspect they kept that to themselves. Their principal concern from the beginning was that I do my best to uncover the truth.

Bibliography

AHPA, CHPA, NNFA, UNPA. Citizens Petition to FDA on Ephedra Labeling. Oct. 25, 2000.

AHPA, CHPA, NNFA, UNPA. Letter to Joe A. Levitt, Oct. 23, 2000.

AHPA, CHPA, CRN, NNFA, UNPA. Letter to Paul M. Coates, Oct 23, 2000.

Armstrong, W. Jeffrey, P. Johnson, and S. Duhme. "The Effect of Commercial Thermogenic Weight Loss Supplement On Body Composition And Energy Expenditure In Obese Adults." *Journal of Exercise Physiology.* 2001: 4(2):28-34.

Avorn, J., M. Chen, and R. Hartley. "Scientific versus commercial sources of influence on the prescribing behavior of physicians." *American Journal of Medicine.* 1982: 73:4-8.

Bell, C., J.M. Kowalchuk, D.H. Paterson, B.W. Scheuermann, and D.A. Cunningham. "The effects of caffeine on the kinetics of O_2 uptake, CO_2 production and expiratory ventilation in humans during the on-transient of moderate and heavy intensity exercise." *Exp Physiol.* 1999: 84(4):761-74.

Bent, S., T.N. Tiedt, M.C Odden, and M.G. Shlipak. "The Relative Safety of Ephedra Compared with Other Herbal products." *Annals of Internal Medicine.* 2003: 138.

Bero, L.A., and D. Rennie. "Influences on the quality of published drug studies." *Int J Technol Assess Health Care.* 1996: 12(2):209-37.

Blumenthal, D., E.G. Campbell, M.S. Anderson, N. Causino, and K.S. Louis. "Withholding research results in academic life science: evidence from a national survey of faculty." *JAMA.* 1997: 277:1224-8.

Boozer, C.N., P.A. Daly, P. Homel, J.L. Solomon, D. Blanchard, J.A Nasser, R. Strauss, and T. Meredith. "Herbal ephedra/caffeine for weight loss: a 6-month randomized safety and efficacy trial." *The International Journal of Obesity.* 2002: 26:593-604.

Boozer, C.N., J.A. Nasser, S.B Heymsfield, V. Wang, G. Chen, and J.L. Solomon. "An herbal supplement containing Ma Huang-Guarana for weight loss: a randomized, double-blind trial." *Int J Obes Relat Metab Disord.* 2001: 25(3):316-24.

Bravo, E. "Phenylpropanolamine and other over-the counter vasoactive compounds." *Hypertension* 1988: 11(SUPPL II):7-10.

Brennan, T.A. "Buying editorials." *N Engl J Med.* 1994: 331:673-5.

Bright, T.P., B.W. Sandage Jr., and H.P. Fletcher. "Selected cardiac and metabolic responses to pseudoephedrine with exercise." *Journal of Clinical Pharmacology* 1981: 21(11-12 Pt 1): 488-92.

Brown, W.A. "Are antidepressants as ineffective as they look?" *Prevention & Treatment.* 2002: 5:Article 26.

Cauchon, D. "FDA advisers tied to industry." *USA Today.* 2000: 1A.

Caudill, T.S., M.S. Johnson, E.C Rich, and W.P. McKinney. "Physicians, pharmaceutical sales representatives, and the cost of prescribing." *Arch of Fam Med.* 1996: 5:201-206.

Chalmers, I. "Underreporting research is scientific misconduct." *JAMA.* 1990: 263:1405-8.

Cho, M.K., R. Shohara, A. Schissel, and D. Rennie. "Policies on faculty conflicts of interest at US universities." *JAMA.* 2000: 284:2203-2208.

Clemons, J.M., and S.L Crosby. "Cardiopulmonary and subjective effects of a 60 mg dose of pseudoephedrine on graded treadmill exercise." *Journal of Sports Medicine and Physical Fitness.* 1993: 33(4):405-12.

Cook, H. "Practical guide to medical education." *Pharmaceutical Marketing.* 2001.

Cox, Teri. Commentary in *Pharma Executive.* September 2002.

Daly, P.A., D.R. Krieger, A.G. Dulloo, J.B. Young, and L. Landsberg. " Ephedrine, caffeine and aspirin: safety and efficacy for treatment of human obesity." *Int J Obesity.* 1993: 17(Supp. 1):S73-S78.

Davidson, Jonathan. et al. "Effect of *Hypericum perforatum* (St John's Wort) in Major Depressive Disorder." *JAMA.* 2002: 287:1807-1814.

Davidson, R.A. "Source of funding and outcome of clinical trials." *Journal of General Internal Medicine.* 1986: 1:155-8.

Davis, R. "Health education on the six-o'clock news. Motivating television coverage of news in medicine." *JAMA* 1988: 259(7):1036-8.

Davis, Ron. "Dangers of Dietary Supplement Ephedra, Statement for the Record of the American Medical Association to the Subcommittee on Oversight of Government Management, Restructuring and the District of Columbia Committee on Government Affairs." United States Senate. October 8, 2002.

Davis, C., and E. Saltos. "Dietary recommendations and how they have changed over time. In: Elizabeth Frazao, America's eating habits: changes and consequences. Washington, DC: U.S. Department of Agriculture, Food and Rural Economics Division." *Agriculture Information Bulletin No. 750.* 1999: p. 33-50.

"Dietary Supplement Industry Calls on FDA to Adopt National Standards on Ephedra." Ephedra Education Council. Oct. 26, 2000.

Dietary Supplements for Weight Loss: Limited Federal Oversight Has Focused More on Marketing than on Safety (Testimony: 07/31/2002, GAO-02-985T).

Dietary Supplements: Uncertainties in Analyses Underlying FDA's Proposed Rule on Ephedrine Alkaloids (Letter Report: 07/02/1999, GAO/ HEHS/GGD).

"Drug Marketing." *The New England Journal of Medicine.* 2002: 346:498-505,524-531.

DiMasi, Joseph et al. "The Cost of Innovation in the Pharmaceutical Industry." *Journal of Health Economics.* 1991: 10:107-142.

Elias, M. "Antidepressant barely better than placebo." *USA Today.* July 7, 2002.

Emerson, Bo. "Chewin' the fat: Whose Fault is Obesity?" *Atlanta Journal and Constitution.* July 5 2003.

Federal Register. March 13, 2003. Vol. 68, No. 49.

Federal Register. Sept. 23, 1997. Vol. 49, p. 838-39.

Fessenden, Ford. "Studies of Dietary Supplements Come Under Growing Scrutiny." *New York Times.* June 23, 2003.

Flanagin, A., L.A. Carey, P.B. Fontanarosa, et al. "Prevalence of articles with honorary authors and ghost authors in peer-reviewed medical journals." *JAMA.* 1998: 280:222-4.

Food and Drug Administration. 62 *Fed. Reg.* 30678, June 4, 1997.

Freemantle, N., I.M. Anderson, and P. Young. "Predictive value of pharmacological activity for the relative efficacy of antidepressant drugs: Meta-regression analysis." 2002. *British Journal of Psychiatry.* 177: 292-302.

Friedberg, M., B. Saffran, T.J. Stinson, W. Nelson, and C.L. Bennett. "Evaluation of conflict of interest in economic analyses of new drugs used in oncology." *JAMA.* 1999: 282:1453-7.

General Accounting Office. "Dietary Supplements: Uncertainties in Analyses Underying FDA's Proposed Rule on Ephedrine Alkaloids." (GAO/HEHS/GGD-99-90). Washington, D.C. *General Accounting Office.* July 2, 1999.

Getz, K.A. "AMCs rekindling clinical research partnerships with industry." *Centerwatch.* 1999.

Gibbons, R.V., Landry, F.J., Blouch, D.L., et al. "A comparison of physicians' and patients' attitudes toward pharmaceutical industry gifts." *JGIM.* 1998: 13:151-154.

Greene, J., Marsden, M., Sanchez, R., et al. "National Household Survey on Drug Abuse—main findings 1998." Rockville, MD: Dept. of Health and Human Services, Substance Abuse and Mental Health Administration, Office of Applied Statistics. 2000: Report No.: H-11.

Greenway, F.L. "The safety and efficacy of pharmaceutical and herbal caffeine and ephedrine use as a weight loss agent." *Obes Rev.* 2001: 2(3):199-211.

Gugliotta, G. "FDA Backs off Former Weight Loss Policy." *Washington Post.* Feb. 29, 2000; Page A02.

"Guidelines for communicating emerging science on nutrition, food safety and health." *J Natl Cancer Inst.* 1998: 90(3):194-9.

Haller, C.A., P. Jacob., and N.L. Benowitz. "Pharmacology of Ephedra Alakaloids and Caffeine After Single-Dose Dietary

Supplement Use." *Clinical Pharmacology and Therapeutics.* 2002: 71(6):421-31.

"How Accurate is the FDA's Monitoring of Supplements Like Ephedra?" Committee on Government Reform. House of Representatives. May 1999.

"Effect of *Hypericum Perforatum* (St John's wort) in major depressive disorder: A randomized controlled trial." Hypericum Depression Trial Study Group. *Journal of the American Medical Association.* 2002: 287:1807-1814.

Jacobson, N.S., L.J. Roberts, S.B. Berns, and J.B. McGlinchey. "Methods defining and determining the clinical significance of treatment effects: Description, application, and alternatives." *Journal of Consulting & Clinical Psychology.* 1999: 67:300-307.

Jones, G. "Interpretation of postmortem drug levels." *Drug Abuse Handbook.* 1998: Boca Raton, Fl: CRC Press: 970-987.

Jones, W.K. "Safety of Dietary Supplements Containing Ephedrine Alkaloids." Office of Women's Health Report on Public Hearing. Aug. 8-9, 2000.

Kaitin, Kenneth I. and Elaine M. Healy, "The New Drug Approvals of 1998, 1997 and 1996: Emerging Drug Development Trends in the User Fee Era," Tufts Center for the Study of Drug Development. January 2000. *PAREXEL's Pharmaceutical R&D Statistical Sourcebook.* p. 117.

Kanfer, I., R. Dowse, V. Vuma. "Pharmacokinetics of oral decongestants." *Pharmacotherapy.* 1993: 13(6 Pt 2):116S-128S,143S-146S.

Kassirer, J.P. "Financial indigestion." *JAMA.* 2000: 284:2156-2157.

Kaufman, D.W., J.P. Kelly, L. Rosenberg, T.E. Anderson, and A.A. Mitchell. "Recent Patterns Of Medication Use in the Ambulatory Adult Population of the United States: The Slone Survey." *JAMA.* 2002: 287(3):337-44.

Kaufman, L. "Prime-time nutrition." *Journal of Communication.* 1990: 30(3):37-45.

Kernan, W.N., C.M. Viscoli, L.M. Brass, J.P. Broderick, T. Brott, et al. "Phenylpropanolamine and the Risk of Hemorrhagic Stroke." *NEJM.* 2000: 343(25):1826-32.

Khan, A., H.A. Warner., and W.A. Brown. "Symptom reduction and suicide risk in patients treated with placebo in antidepressant clinical trials: An analysis of the Food and Drug Administration database." *Archives of General Psychiatry.* 2000: 57:311-317.

Kissin, W., T. Garfield, and J. Ball. "Drug Abuse Warning Network." Annual Medical Examiner data. Bethesda: Dept. of Health and Human Services, Substance Abuse and Mental Health Administration, Office of Applied Statistics. 2000: Report No.: D-13.

Kissin, W., T. Garfield, and J. Ball. "Mid-year 1999 preliminary emergency department data from the Drug Abuse Warning Network." D-14. Bethesda: Dept. of Health and Human Services. Substance Abuse and Mental Health Administration. Office of Applied Statistics. 2000.

Korn, D. "Conflicts of interest in biomedical research." *JAMA.* 2000: 284:2234-2237.

Kunin, C.M. "Clinical investigators and the pharmaceutical industry." *Ann Intern Med.* 1978: 89(Suppl):842-5.

Levy, D. "Ghostwriters a hidden resource for drug makers." *USA Today.* September 25, 1996.

Lexchin, J. "What information do physicians receive from pharmaceutical representatives?" *Can Fam Phys.* 1997: 43:941-945.

Lutz, Katherine. "Can a Popular Antidepressant Cause Teenage Suicide?" *Boston Globe.* August 5, 2003.

McNamara, Stephen H., and Wes A. Siegner. "FDA Has Substantial and Sufficient Authority to Regulate Dietary Supplements" *Food & Drug Law Inastitute.* 2002: 57:15-24.

Morgenstern, L.B., C.M. Viscoli, W.N. Kernan, L.M. Brass, J.P. Broderick, E. Feldmann, et al. "Use of Ephedra-Containing Products and Risk for Hemorrhagic Stroke." *Neurology.* 2003: 60(1):132-5.

Morton, R.H. "Effects of caffeine, ephedrine and their combinations on time to exhaustion during high-intensity exercise." *European Journal of Applied Physiology.* 1999: 79(4):379-81.

Nelkin, D. "An uneasy relationship: the tensions between medicine and the media." *Lancet.* 1996: 347(9015):1600-3.

"Off the Charts: Pay, Profits, and Spending by Drug Companies." *Families USA.* Pub No. 01-104.

"The Pharmaceutical Industry Into Its Second Century: From Serendipity to Strategy." Boston Consulting Group. January 1999. pgs 51-56.

"Pharmaceutical R&D: Costs, Risks and Rewards." Office of Technology Assessment, U.S. Congress. 1993.

Oral Testimony of the Consumer Healthcare Products Association, to the White House Commission on Complementary and Alternative Medicine Policy. Minnesota Town Hall Meeting. March 16, 2001.

Peterson, M. "What's black and white and sells medicine?" *New York Times*. August 27, 2000: sect 3:1.

"Prescription Drugs and Mass Media Advertising." The National Institute for Health Care Management Foundation. 2001.

"Prescription Drug Expenditures in 2000: The Upward Trend Continues." The National Institute for Health Care Management Foundation. May 2001.

"The Relation between Voluntary Notification and Material Risk in Dietary Supplement Safety." *FDA Docket*. 2000: 00N-1200(41).

Rennie, D., and A. Flanagin. "Authorship! Authorship! Guests, ghosts, grafters, and the two-sided coin." *JAMA*. 1994: 271:469-71.

"Report of the Advisory Review Panel on OTC cold, cough, allergy, bronchodilator, and antiasthmatic products." *Federal Register*. 1976: 41:38403.

Rochon, P.A., J.H. Gurwitz, R.W. Simms, et al. "A study of manufacturer-supported trials of nonsteroidal anti-inflammatory drugs in the treatment of arthritis." *Arch Intern Med*. 1994: 154:157-63.

"Safety Assessment and Determination of a Tolerable Upper Limit for Ephedra." CANTOX Report on Ephedra. CANTOX Health Sciences International. 2000.

Samenuk, D., M.S. Link, M.K. Homoud, R. Contreras, T.C. Theohardes, P.J. Wang, N.A. Estes. "Adverse Cardiovascular Events Temporally Associated with Ma Huang, an Herbal Source of Ephedrine." *Mayo Clinic Proceedings*. 2002: 77(1):12-6.

Sensenbrenner, F. James. "GAO Report Questions Science Behind FDA's Action on Ephedrine Alkaloids." Committee on Science. August 4, 1999.

Siegner, Wes A. "New laws are not needed." *USA Today*. July 16, 2003.

Shekelle, P.G., M.L. Hardy, M. Maglione, and S.C. Morton. "Ephedra and Ephedrine for Weight Loss and Athletic Performance Enhancement: Clinical Efficacy and Side Effects." Agency for

Healthcare Research and Quality. 2002.

Suissa, S., P. Ernst, J.F. Boivin, R.I. Horwitz, B. Habbick, D. Cockroft, et al. "A cohort analysis of excess mortality in asthma and the use of inhaled beta-agonists." *Am J Respir Crit Care Med.* 1994: 149:604.

Swain, R.A., D.M Harsha, J. Baenziger, R.M. Saywell Jr. "Do pseudoephedrine or phenylpropanolamine improve maximum oxygen uptake and time to exhaustion?" *Clin J Sport Med.* 1997: 7(3):168-73.

Taylor, H., and R. Leitman, eds. "Widespread Ignorance of Regulation and Labeling of Vitamins, Minerals and Food Supplements, According to a National Harris Interactive Survey." *Harris Interactive Health Care News.* 2002: 2(23):1-5.

"Tylenol Deaths." *Journal of Pediatrics.* 1998: 132.

Vahedi, K., V. Domigo, P. Amarenco, and M.G. Bousser MG. "Ischaemic stroke in a sportsman who consumed MaHuang extract and creatine monohydrate for body building." *J Neurol Neurosurg Psychiatry.* 2000: 68(1):112-3.

Vansal, S.S., and D.R. Feller. "Direct effects of ephedrine isomers on human beta-adrenergic receptor subtypes." *Biochemical Pharmacology* 1999: 58(5):807-10.

Walker, A. "The Relation between Voluntary Notification and Material Risk in Dietary Supplement Safety." *FDA Docket.* 2000: 00N-1200.

Wazana, A. "Physicians and the Pharmaceutical Industry: Is a gift ever just a gift?" *JAMA.* 2000: 283, No 3.

White, L.M., S.F. Gardner, B.J. Gurley, M.A. Marx, P.L Wang, and M. Estes. "Pharmacokinetics and cardiovascular effects of ma-huang (Ephedra sinica) in normotensive adults." *J Clin Pharmacol.* 1997: 37(2):116-22.

Wolfe, Sidney M. "Ephedra Scientific Evidence Versus Money/Politics." *Science.* April 19, 2003.

Wolfe, S,M. "Why do American drug companies spend more than $12 billion a year pushing drugs? Is it education or promotion?" *J of Gen Int Med.* 1996: 11:637-9.

Wood, A.J.J., C.M. Stein, and R. Woosley. "Making medicines safer— the need for an independent drug safety board." *N Engl J Med.* 1998: 339:1851-4.

Books

Bian, Tonda R. *The Drug Lords: America's Pharmaceutical Cartel.* No Barriers Pub: 1997.

Chang, H.M. and P.P.H. But. *Pharmacology and Applications of Chinese Materia Medica.* World Scientific: 1986.

Cohen, Jay. *Over Dose: The Case Against the Drug Companies: Prescription Drugs, Side Effects, and Your Health.* Penguin USA: 2001.

Fried, Stephen M. *Bitter Pills: Inside the Hazardous World of Legal Drugs.* Bantam Doubleday Dell: 1998.

Greider, Katharine. *The Big Fix: How the Pharmaceutical Industry Rips Off American Consumers.* Public Affairs: 2003.

Hawthorne, Fran. *The Merck Druggernaut: The Inside Story of a Pharmaceutical Giant.* John Wiley & Sons: 2003.

Higgs, Robert (ed), Ronald W. Hansen, Paul H. Rubin. *Hazardous to Our Health? FDA Regulation of Health Care Products.* Independent Institute: 1995.

Hilts, Philip J. *Protecting America's Health: The Fda, Business, and One Hundred Years of Regulation.* Knopf: 2003.

Huang, K.C. *The Pharmacology of Chinese Herbs.* CRC Press: 1993.

Marsa, Linda. *Prescription for Profits: How the Pharmaceutical Industry Bankrolled the Unholy Marriage Between Science and Business.* Scribner: 1999.

Miller, Henry I., John J. Cohrssen, and Terry L. Anderson. *To America's Health: A Proposal to Reform the Food and Drug Administration.* Hoover Institution Press Publication: 2000.

Moore, Thomas J. *Deadly Medicine: Why Tens of Thousands of Heart Patients Died in America'a Worst Drug Disaster.* Simon & Schuster: 1995.

Mundy, Alicia. *Dispensing With the Truth: The Victims, the Drug Companies, and the Dramatic Story Behind the Battle over Fen-Phen.* St. Martin's Press: 2001.

Papas, Andreas M., and Jean Carper. *The Vitamin E Factor: The Miraculous Antioxidant for the Prevention and Treatment of Heart Disease, Cancer, and Aging.* HarperCollins: 1999.

Stauber, John, and Sheldon Rampton. *Trust Us We're Experts: How*

Industry Manipulates Science and Gambles with Your Future. J.P. Tarcher: 2002.

Tang, W. and G. Eisenbrand. *Chinese Drugs of Plant Origin.* Springer-Verlag: 1992.

Websites

American Botanical Council
www.herbalgram.org

American Council on Science and Health (ACSH)
www.acsh.org

American Obesity Association
www.obesity.org

Centers for Disease Control and Prevention
www.cdc.gov

Center For Consumer Freedom (CCF)
www.CCF.org

Center for Media & Democracy (PR Watch)
www.prwatch.org

The Center for Public Integrity
www.publicintegrity.org/dtaweb/home.asp

Council for Responsible Nutrition
www.crnusa.org

Center for Science in the Public Interest (CSPI)
www.cspinet.org

Ephedra Education Council
www.ephedrafacts.com

FDA News
www.fda.gov/opacom/hpwhats.html

FDA Conflicts of Interest web page
www.lasikinfocenter.net/Webpages/FDA%20Conflicts%20of%20Int
  erest%20Webpage.htm

FDA Review.Org—A Project of the Independent Institute
www.fdareview.org/glossary.shtml#elixir

Food and Nutrition Board (FNB) of the National Academy of Sciences
www.iom.edu/IOM/IOMHome.nsf/Pages/About+FNB

Food Policy Institute at the Consumer Federation of America
www.consumerfed.org

Harvard School of Public Health Nutrition Source
www.hsph.harvard.edu/nutritionsource

International Food Information Council Foundation (IFIC)
www.ific.org/food

Steven Milloy
www.JunkScience.com

National Advisory Council for Complementary and Alternative
  Medicine (NACCAM)
nccam.nih.gov

National Food Processors Association
www.nfpa-food.org

National Institutes of Health
www.nih.gov

Office of Dietary Supplements, National Institutes of Health
www.dietary-supplements.info.nih.gov

PharmaVoice
www.pharmalinx.com

The Pharmaceutical Research and Manufacturers of America
  (PhRMA)
www.phrma.org

Physicians Committee for Responsible Medicine
www.pcrm.org

Public Citizen
www.citizen.org

QuackWatch
www.quackwatch.com

Rand Report
www.fda.gov/OHRMS/DOCKETS/98fr/95n-0304-bkg0003
-ref-07-01-index.htm

RxPolicy: PhRMA Watch
www.rxpolicy.com/phrma.html

University of California Berkeley's Wellness Letter
www.berkeleywellness.com

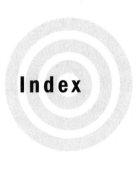

Index

About the Author

Mike Fillon has written about health and medical topics for more than 15 years. For *Popular Mechanics,* he has written over 400 articles on a broad variety of medical, technological, and scientific subjects. Recently he wrote six cover stories—including two articles for two of the top-selling issues in the magazine's 100-year history. Mr. Fillon has written more than 150 consumer-oriented news and feature stories for WebMD, CBS HealthWatch, MSNBC, and the *Reader's Digest* Web sites. He has written both short and feature-length pieces for more than two dozen other publications, including *Health Week, NCN News*—a Novartis Pharmaceutical newsletter—*Information Week* and *Science Digest.* He has also written for the American Cancer Society, Emory University and the Center for Disease Control and Prevention (CDC). Additionally, he has been interviewed on numerous radio shows and has appeared on the *Weekend Today Show* and *American Morning* with Paula Zahn.

Mr. Fillon has recently published two very successful health booklets: *Conquering Caffeine Dependence* and *Conquering Food Triggers.* He also had two books published in 1999: *Natural Prostate Healers,* by Prentice Hall, and *Young Superstars of Tennis,* for Avisson Press. He also contributed a number of chapters for the *Reader's Digest* title *Looking After Your Body.* He wrote sections on shingles, problems of the gall bladder, thyroid, prostate, back problems, and a wide range of gastrointestinal illnesses.

Mr. Fillon has a Master of Science degree of the State University of New York Maritime College. He is a member of the American Medical Writer's Association and the National Association of Science Writers.

Mr. Fillon lives in Atlanta with his wife, Sue, their children Sarah, Emilie and Evan, and a golden retriever named Sandy Koufax.

Do You Have an Opinion about ephedra or your rights to vitamins, minerals, herbs and other dietary supplements? If so, contact your representative and let them know how you feel:

United States House of Representatives

write: U.S. House of Representatives
Washington, D.C. 20515

phone: (202) 225-3121

on the web: http://www.house.gov

United States Senate

write: U.S. Senate
Hart Senate Office Building
Washington, D.C. 20510

               U.S. Senate
Dirksen Senate Office Building
Washington, D.C. 20510

               U.S. Senate
Russell Senate Office Building
Washington, D.C. 20510

phone: (202) 224-3121

on the web: http://www.senate.gov